MICROWAVE COOKBOOK 2022

TASTY HOMEMADE RECIPES IN MINUTES FOR BEGINNERS

VERONICA WOODS

Table of Contents

Braised Beef and Vegetables *15*
Beef Stew *16*
Beef and Vegetable Hot-pot *17*
Beef Curry *18*
Basic Mince *19*
Cottage Pie *20*
Cottage Pie with Cheese *20*
Mince with Oats *21*
Chilli con Carne *21*
Curried Mince *22*
Beef Goulash *23*
Beef Goulash with Boiled Potatoes *24*
Butter Bean and Beef Stew with Tomatoes *24*
Beef and Tomato Cake *25*
Beef and Mushroom Kebabs *26*
Stuffed Lamb *28*
Minted Lamb Kebabs *29*
Classic Lamb Kebabs *30*
Middle Eastern Lamb with Fruit *31*
Mock Irish Stew *32*
Farmer's Wife Lamb Chops *33*
Lamb Hot-pot *34*

Lamb Loaf with Mint and Rosemary	35
Lamb Bredie with Tomatoes	36
Lamb Biriani	37
Ornate Biriani	38
Moussaka	39
Moussaka with Potatoes	40
Quick Moussaka	41
Lamb Mince	42
Shepherd's Pie	42
Country Liver in Red Wine	43
Liver and Bacon	44
Liver and Bacon with Apple	45
Kidneys in Red Wine with Brandy	46
Venison Steaks with Oyster Mushrooms and Blue Cheese	48
Cooking Small Pasta	49
Chinese Noodle and Mushroom Salad with Walnuts	49
Pepper Macaroni	50
Family Macaroni Cheese	51
Classic Macaroni Cheese	52
Macaroni Cheese with Stilton	53
Macaroni Cheese with Bacon	53
Macaroni Cheese with Tomatoes	53
Spaghetti Carbonara	54
Pizza-style Macaroni Cheese	55
Spaghetti Cream with Spring Onions	56
Spaghetti Bolognese	57
Spaghetti with Turkey Bolognese Sauce	58

Spaghetti with Ragu Sauce 59
Spaghetti with Butter 60
Pasta with Garlic 61
Spaghetti with Beef and Mixed Vegetable Bolognese Sauce 62
Spaghetti with Meat Sauce and Cream 63
Spaghetti with Marsala Meat Sauce 63
Pasta alla Marinara 64
Pasta Matriciana 65
Pasta with Tuna and Capers 66
Pasta Napoletana 67
Pasta Pizzaiola 68
Pasta with Peas 68
Pasta with Chicken Liver Sauce 68
Pasta with Anchovies 69
Ravioli with Sauce 69
Tortellini 70
Lasagne 71
Pizza Napoletana 72
Pizza Margherita 73
Seafood Pizza 73
Pizza Siciliana 73
Mushroom Pizza 73
Ham and Pineapple Pizza 74
Pepperoni Pizzas 74
Buttered Flaked Almonds 75
Flaked Almonds in Garlic Butter 75
Dried Chestnuts 75

Drying Herbs	76
Crisping Breadcrumbs	77
Nut Burgers	78
Nutkin Cake	79
Buckwheat	80
Bulgar	81
Bulgar with Fried Onion	82
Tabbouleh	83
Sultan's Salad	84
Couscous	85
Grits	86
Gnocchi alla Romana	87
Ham Gnocchi	88
Millet	89
Polenta	90
Grilled Polenta	91
Polenta with Pesto	91
Polenta with Sun-dried Tomato or Olive Paste	91
Quinoa	92
Romanian Polenta	93
Curried Rice	94
Cottage Cheese and Rice Casserole	95
Italian Risotto	96
Mushroom Risotto	97
Brazilian Rice	97
Spanish Rice	98
Plain Turkish Pilaf	99

Rich Turkish Pilaf	100
Thai Rice with Lemon Grass, Lime Leaves and Coconut	101
Okra with Cabbage	102
Red Cabbage with Apple	103
Red Cabbage with Wine	105
Norwegian Sour Cabbage	105
Greek-style Stewed Okra with Tomatoes	106
Greens with Tomatoes, Onions and Peanut Butter	107
Sweet-sour Creamed Beetroot	108
Beetroot in Orange	109
Scalloped Celeriac	110
Celeriac with Orange Hollandaise Sauce	111
Slimmers' Vegetable Pot	112
Slimmers' Vegetable Pot with Eggs	112
Ratatouille	113
Caramelised Parsnips	114
Parsnips with Egg and Butter Crumb Sauce	115
Chocolate Fondue	116
Orange Chocolate Fondue	116
Mocha Fondue	117
White Chocolate Fondue	117
Toblerone Fondue	117
Royal Chocolate Mousse	118
Dutch-style Pears with Chocolate Advocaat Mousse	119
Traditional Chocolate Mousse	120
Chocolate Orange Mousse	120
Mocha Mousse	121

Chocolate Peppermint Cream Mousse	*121*
Berlin Air	*122*
Crème Caramel	*123*
Spicy Peaches and Oranges in Red Wine	*123*
Spicy Pears and Oranges in Red Wine	*124*
Store-cupboard Raspberry Mousse	*125*
Egg Custard, Apricot and Sherry Trifle	*126*
Short-cut Sherry Trifle	*128*
Chocolate Cream Trifle	*129*
Trifle with Sponge Cakes	*129*
Fluffy Lemon Clouds	*130*
Fluffy Lime Clouds	*131*
Apple Snow	*131*
Apricot Snow	*132*
Lemon Meringue Spiced Pears	*133*
Finnish Cranberry Whip	*134*
Cranberry and Orange Whip	*135*
Kissel	*136*
Home-made Yoghurt	*137*
Apricot Pots	*138*
Prune Pots	*139*
Cherries Jubilee	*140*
Fruits of the Forest Jubilee	*140*
Dutch Chocolate Sundaes	*141*
Cream Liqueur Sundaes	*141*
Grape and Raspberry Jelly	*142*
Mandarin and Lemon Jelly	*142*

Black Cherry Rice Cream 143
Banana Splits 143
Spicy Prune Froth 144
Chilled Oranges with Hot Chocolate Peppermint Sauce 145
Summer Fruit Mould 145
Watermelon and Apricot Chill with Frosted Grapes 146
Rhubarb and Mandarin Cups 147
Rhubarb and Mandarin Cups with Ginger Cream 148
Chocolate Strawberries on Pineapple Sorbet 149
Danish Apple 'Cake' 150
Peasant Girl with Veil 151
Imperial Rice 152
Children's Fruity Mousse 153
Raspberry and Blackcurrant Mousse 154
Welsh Rarebit 155
Mixed Cheese Rarebit 155
Buck Rarebit 156
Bacon Rarebit 156
Beer Rarebit 157
Open-topped Hungarian Salami Sandwiches 158
Granola 159
Honey Granola 160
Porridge 160
Bacon 161
Basic White Sauce 162
Béchamel Sauce 163
Caper Sauce 164

Cheese Sauce 164

Mornay Sauce 164

Egg Sauce 165

Mushroom Sauce 165

Mustard Sauce 165

Onion Sauce 166

Parsley Sauce 166

Watercress Sauce 166

Pouring Sauce 167

All-in-one Sauce 167

Hollandaise Sauce 168

Short-cut Béarnaise Sauce 169

Maltese Sauce 169

Mayonnaise Sauce 170

Cocktail Sauce 171

Louis Sauce 171

Thousand Island Dressing 173

Green Sauce 174

Rémoulade Sauce 174

Sauce Tartare 175

No-egg Mayonnaise-style Dressing 175

Mint Sauce 176

Orange Sauce 176

Jellied Mixed Herb Sauce 177

Jellied Herb Sauce with Lemon 178

Salsa 178

Smooth Salsa 179

Extra-hot Salsa	179
Coriander Salsa	179
Apple Sauce	180
Mrs Beeton's Brown Apple Sauce	180
Gooseberry Sauce	181
Salsa with Sweetcorn	182
Austrian Apple and Horseradish Sauce	183
Garlic Sauce	184
Apple and Horseradish Sauce	185
Bread Sauce	186
Brown Bread Sauce	187
Cranberry Sauce	187
Cranberry Wine Sauce	188
Cranberry Orange Sauce	188
Cranberry and Apple Sauce	188
Cumberland Sauce	189
Slovenian Wine Sauce	190
Thin Gravy for Poultry	191
Thick Gravy for Meat	192
Short-cut Oriental Sauce	192
Indonesian-style Peanut Sauce	193
Creole Sauce	194
Quick Creole Sauce	195
Newburg Sauce	196
Piquant Brown Sauce	197
Piquant Sauce with Pickled Walnuts	198
Portuguese Sauce	198

Rustic Tomato Sauce	200
Curried Turkey Sauce for Jacket Potatoes	201
Tandoori Turkey Sauce for Jacket Potatoes	202
Hot Chilli Beef Sauce for Jacket Potatoes	202
Chop House Sauce	203
Hot Cheese and Carrot Sauce for Jacket Potatoes	204
Basting Sauces	205
Butter Baste	205
Spicy Curry Baste	206
Jalapeno Mexican Barbecue Baste	206
Tomato Baste	207
Dutch Butter Blender Cream	208
Dutch Butter Blender Cream with Vanilla	208
Hot Chocolate Sauce	209
Mocha Sauce	209
Hot Chocolate and Orange Sauce	210
Hot Chocolate Peppermint Sauce	210
Raspberry Coulis	210
Summer Fruit Coulis	211
Apricot Coulis	212
Home-made Caramel Sauce	213
Egg Custard Sauce	214
Flavoured Egg Custard Sauce	215
Lemon or Orange Custard	215
Brandy Sauce	215
Rum Sauce	216
Orange Sauce	216

Sticky Toffee Sauce *217*
Fresh Raspberry Sauce *217*
Chocolate Honey Raisin Sauce...*218*

Braised Beef and Vegetables

Serves 4

30 ml/2 tbsp butter or margarine, at kitchen temperature
1 large onion, grated
3 carrots, thinly sliced
75 g/3 oz mushrooms, thinly sliced
450 g/1 lb rump (tip) steak, cut into small cubes
1 beef stock cube
15 ml/1 tbsp plain (all-purpose) flour
300 ml/½ pt/1¼ cups hot water or beef stock
Freshly ground black pepper
5 ml/1 tsp salt

Put the butter or margarine into a 20 cm/8 in diameter casserole dish (Dutch oven). Melt on Defrost for 45 seconds. Add the vegetables and steak and mix well. Cook, uncovered, on Full for 3 minutes. Crumble in the stock cube and stir in the flour and hot water or stock. Move the mixture to the edge of the dish to form a ring, leaving a small hollow in the centre. Sprinkle with pepper. Cover with clingfilm (plastic wrap) and slit it twice to allow steam to escape. Cook on Full for 9 minutes, turning the dish once. Allow to stand for 5 minutes, then season with the salt and serve.

Beef Stew

Serves 4

450 g/1 lb lean stewing steak, cut into small cubes
15 ml/1 tbsp plain (all-purpose) flour
250 g/9 oz unthawed frozen vegetable stewpack
300 ml/½ pt/1¼ cups boiling water
1 beef stock cube
Freshly ground pepper
2.5–5 ml/½–1 tsp salt

Put the steak in a 23 cm/9 in diameter casserole dish (Dutch oven), not too deep. Sprinkle with the flour, then toss well to coat. Spread out loosely into a single layer. Break up the vegetables, then arrange round the meat. Cover with clingfilm (plastic wrap) and slit it twice to allow steam to escape. Cook on Full for 15 minutes, turning the dish four times. Pour the water over the meat and crumble in the stock cube. Season to taste with pepper and stir thoroughly. Cover as before, then cook on Full for 10 minutes, turning the dish three times. Allow to stand for 5 minutes, then stir round, season with the salt and serve.

Beef and Vegetable Hot-pot

Serves 4

450 g/1 lb potatoes

2 carrots

1 large onion

450 g/1 lb lean stewing steak, cut into small cubes

1 beef stock cube

150 ml/¼ pt/2/3 cup hot beef or vegetable stock

30 ml/2 tbsp butter or margarine

Cut the potatoes, carrots and the onion into transparent wafer-thin slices. Separate the onion slices into rings. Thoroughly grease a 1.75 litre/3 pt/7½ cup dish. Fill with alternate layers of the vegetables and meat, beginning and ending with the potatoes. Cover with clingfilm (plastic wrap) and slit it twice to allow steam to escape. Cook on Full for 15 minutes, turning the dish three times. Crumble the stock cube into the hot stock and stir until dissolved. Pour gently down the side of the dish so it flows through the meat and vegetables. Top with flakes of the butter or margarine. Cover as before and cook on Full for 15 minutes, turning the dish three times. Allow to stand for 5 minutes. Brown under a hot grill (broiler), if liked.

Beef Curry

Serves 4–5

An Anglicised version of a medium-hot curry. Serve with basmati rice and sambals (side dishes) of plain yoghurt, sliced cucumber sprinkled with chopped fresh coriander (cilantro), and chutney.

450 g/1 lb lean stewing beef, cut into small cubes
2 onions, chopped
2 garlic cloves, crushed
15 ml/1 tbsp sunflower or corn oil
30 ml/2 tbsp hot curry powder
30 ml/2 tbsp tomato purée (paste)
15 ml/1 tbsp plain (all-purpose) flour
4 green cardamom pods
15 ml/1 tbsp garam masala
450 ml/¾ pt/2 cups hot water
5 ml/1 tsp salt

Arrange the meat in a single layer in a deep 25 cm/10 in diameter dish. Cover with a plate and cook on Full for 15 minutes, stirring twice. Meanwhile, fry (sauté) the onions and garlic conventionally in the oil in a frying pan (skillet) over a medium heat until pale golden. Stir in the curry powder, tomato purée, flour, cardamom pods and garam masala, then gradually blend in the hot water. Cook, stirring, until the mixture comes to the boil and thickens. Remove the dish of meat from the microwave and stir in the contents of the frying pan. Cover with clingfilm (plastic wrap) and slit it twice to allow steam to escape. Cook on Full for 10 minutes, turning the dish twice. Allow to stand for 5 minutes before serving.

Basic Mince

Serves 4

450 g/1 lb/4 cups lean minced (ground) beef
1 onion, grated
30 ml/2 tbsp plain (all-purpose) flour
450 ml/¾ pt/2 cups hot water
1 beef stock cube
5 ml/1 tsp salt

Place the meat in a deep 20 cm/8 in diameter dish. Thoroughly mix in the onion and flour with a fork. Cook, uncovered, on Full for 5 minutes. Break up the meat with a fork. Add the water and crumble in the stock cube. Stir well to mix. Cover with clingfilm (plastic wrap) and slit it twice to allow steam to escape. Cook on Full for 15 minutes, turning the dish four times. Allow to stand for 4 minutes. Add the salt and stir round before serving.

Cottage Pie

Serves 4

1 quantity Basic Mince
675 g/1½ lb freshly cooked potatoes
30 ml/2 tbsp butter or margarine
60–90 ml/4–6 tbsp hot milk

Cool the Basic Mince to lukewarm and transfer to a greased 1 litre/1¾ pt/4¼ cup pie dish. Cream the potatoes with the butter or margarine and enough of the milk to make a light and fluffy mash. Pipe over the meat mixture or spread smoothly then rough up with a fork. Reheat, uncovered, on Full for 3 minutes. Alternatively, brown under a hot grill (broiler).

Cottage Pie with Cheese

Serves 4

Prepare as for Cottage Pie, but add 50–75 g/2–3 oz/½–¾ cup grated Cheddar cheese to the potatoes after creaming with the butter and hot milk.

Mince with Oats

Serves 4

Prepare as for Basic Mince, but add 1 carrot, grated, with the onion. Substitute 25 g/1 oz/½ cup porridge oats for the flour. Cook for the first time for 7 minutes.

Chilli con Carne

Serves 4–5

450 g/1 lb/4 cups lean minced (ground) beef
1 onion, grated
2 garlic cloves, crushed
5–20 ml/1–4 tsp chilli seasoning
400 g/14 oz/1 large can chopped tomatoes
5 ml/1 tsp Worcestershire sauce
400 g/14 oz/1 large can red kidney beans, drained
5 ml/1 tsp salt
Jacket Potatoes or boiled rice, to serve

Put the beef into a 23 cm/9 in diameter casserole dish (Dutch oven). Stir in the onion and garlic with a fork. Cook, uncovered, on Full for 5 minutes. Break up the meat with a fork. Work in all the remaining ingredients except the salt. Cover with clingfilm (plastic wrap) and slit it twice to allow steam to escape. Cook on Full for 15 minutes, turning the dish three times. Allow to stand for 4 minutes. Season with the salt before serving with jacket potatoes or boiled rice.

Curried Mince

Serves 4

2 onions, grated
2 garlic cloves, crushed
450 g/1 lb/4 cups lean minced (ground) beef
15 ml/1 tbsp plain (all-purpose) flour
5–10 ml/1–2 tbsp mild curry powder
30 ml/2 tbsp fruity chutney
60 ml/4 tbsp tomato purée (paste)
300 ml/½ pt/1¼ cups boiling water
1 beef stock cube
Salt and freshly ground black pepper

Mash together the onions, garlic and beef. Spread into a 20 cm/8 in diameter casserole dish (Dutch oven). Form into a ring round the edge of the dish, leaving small hollow in the centre. Cover with plate and cook on Full for 5 minutes. Break up with fork. Work in the flour, curry powder, chutney and tomato purée. Gradually stir in the water, then crumble in the stock cube. Cover with clingfilm (plastic wrap) and slit it twice to allow steam to escape. Cook on Full for 15 minutes, turning the dish three times. Allow to stand for 4 minutes. Season to taste, then stir round and serve.

Beef Goulash

Serves 6

40 g/1½ oz/3 tbsp butter, margarine or lard
675 g/1½ lb stewing steak, cut into small cubes
2 large onions, grated
1 medium green (bell) pepper, seeded and finely diced
2 garlic cloves, crushed
4 tomatoes, blanched, skinned and chopped
45 ml/3 tbsp tomato purée (paste)
15 ml/1 tbsp paprika
5 ml/1 tsp caraway seeds
5 ml/1 tsp salt
300 ml/½ pt/1¼ cups boiling water
150 ml/¼ pt/2/3 cup soured (dairy sour) cream

Put the fat in a 1.75 litre/3 pt/7½ cup dish. Melt, uncovered, on Full for 1 minute. Mix in the meat, onions, peppers and garlic. Cover with clingfilm (plastic wrap) and slit it twice to allow steam to escape. Cook on Full for 15 minutes, turning the dish four times. Uncover and stir in the tomatoes, tomato purée, paprika and caraway seeds. Cover as before and cook on Full for 15 minutes, turning the dish four times. Season with the salt and gently mix in the boiling water. Ladle into deep plates and top each generously with the cream.

Beef Goulash with Boiled Potatoes

Serves 6

Prepare as for Beef Goulash, but omit the cream and add 2–3 whole boiled potatoes to each serving.

Butter Bean and Beef Stew with Tomatoes

Serves 6

425 g/15 oz/1 large can butter beans
275 g/10 oz/1 can tomato soup
30 ml/2 tbsp dried onions
6 slices braising steak, about 125 g/4 oz each, beaten flat
Salt and freshly ground black pepper

Combine the beans, soup and onions in a 20 cm/8 in diameter casserole dish (Dutch oven). Cover with a plate and cook on Full for 6 minutes, stirring three times. Arrange the steaks round the edge of the dish. Cover with clingfilm (plastic wrap) and slit it twice to allow steam to escape. Cook on Full for 17 minutes, turning the dish three times. Allow to stand for 5 minutes. Uncover and season to taste before serving.

Beef and Tomato Cake

Serves 2–3

275 g/10 oz/2½ cups minced (ground) beef
30 ml/2 tbsp plain (all-purpose) flour
1 egg
5 ml/1 tsp onion powder
150 ml/¼ pt/2/3 cup tomato juice
5 ml/1 tsp soy sauce
5 ml/1 tsp dried oregano
Boiled pasta, to serve

Thoroughly grease a 900 ml/1½ pt/3¾ cup oval pie dish. Mix the beef with all remaining ingredients and spread smoothly into the dish. Cover with clingfilm (plastic wrap) and slit it twice to allow steam to escape. Cook on Full for 7 minutes, turning the dish twice. Allow to stand for 5 minutes. Cut into two or three portions and serve hot with pasta.

Beef and Mushroom Kebabs

Serves 4

24 fresh or dried bay leaves
½ red (bell) pepper, cut into small squares
½ green (bell) pepper, cut into small squares
750 g/1½ lb grilling (broiling) steak, trimmed and cut into 2.5 cm/1 in cubes
175 g/6 oz button mushrooms
50 g/2 oz/¼ cup butter or margarine, at kitchen temperature
5 ml/1 tsp paprika
5 ml/1 tsp Worcestershire sauce
1 garlic clove, crushed
175 g/6 oz/1½ cups rice, boiled

If using dried bay leaves, place in a small dish, add 90 ml/6 tbsp water and cover with a saucer. Heat on Full for 2 minutes to soften. Put the pepper squares into a dish and just cover with water. Cover with a plate and heat on Full for 1 minute to soften. Drain the peppers and bay leaves. Thread the beef, mushrooms, pepper squares and bay leaves on to twelve 10 cm/4 in wooden skewers. Arrange the kebabs like the spokes of a wheel in a deep 25 cm/10 in diameter dish. Put the butter or margarine, paprika, Worcestershire sauce and garlic in a small dish and heat, uncovered, on Full for 1 minute. Brush over the kebabs. Cook, uncovered, on Full for 8 minutes, turning the dish four times. Carefully turn the kebabs over and brush with the rest of the butter mixture. Cook on Full for a further 4 minutes, turning the dish twice. Arrange on a bed of rice and coat with the juices from the dish. Allow three kebabs per person.

Stuffed Lamb

Serves 4

A slightly Middle Eastern approach here. Serve the lamb with warm pitta bread and a green salad dotted with olives and capers.

4 pieces neck of lamb fillet, about 15 cm/6 in long and 675 g/½ lb each
3 large slices white bread with crusts, cubed
1 onion, cut into 6 wedges
45 ml/3 tbsp toasted pine nuts
30 ml/2 tbsp currants
2.5 ml/½ tsp salt
150 g/5 oz/2/3 cup thick Greek plain yoghurt
Ground cinnamon
8 button mushrooms
15 ml/1 tbsp olive oil

Trim the fat from the lamb. Make a lengthways slit in each piece, taking care not to cut right through the meat. Grind up the bread cubes and onion pieces together in a food processor or blender. Scrape out into a bowl and mix in the pine nuts, currants and salt. Spread equal amounts into the lamb pieces and secure with wooden cocktail sticks (toothpicks). Arrange in a square in a deep 25 cm/10 in diameter dish. Smear with all the yoghurt and dust lightly with cinnamon. Stud randomly with the mushrooms and coat thinly with the oil. Cover with clingfilm (plastic wrap) and slit it twice to allow steam to escape.

Cook on Full for 16 minutes, turning the dish four times. Allow to stand for 5 minutes, then serve.

Minted Lamb Kebabs

Serves 6

900 g/2 lb neck of lamb fillet, trimmed
12 large mint leaves
60 ml/4 tbsp thick plain yoghurt
60 ml/4 tbsp tomato ketchup (catsup)
1 garlic clove, crushed
5 ml/1 tsp Worcestershire sauce
6 pitta breads, warmed
Lettuce leaves, tomato and cucumber slices

Cut the meat into 2.5 cm/1 in cubes. Thread on to six wooden skewers alternately with the mint leaves. Arrange like the spokes of a wheel in a deep 25 cm/10 in diameter dish. Thoroughly combine the yoghurt, ketchup, garlic and Worcestershire sauce and brush half the mixture over the kebabs. Cook, uncovered, on Full for 8 minutes, turning the dish twice. Turn the kebabs over and brush with the remaining baste. Cook on Full for a further 8 minutes, turning the dish twice. Allow to stand for 5 minutes. Warm the pitta breads briefly under the grill (broiler) until they puff up, then slice along the long edge to make a pocket. Remove the meat from the skewers and discard the bay leaves. Pack the lamb into the pittas, then add a good helping of the salad to each.

Classic Lamb Kebabs

Serves 6

900 g/2 lb neck of lamb fillet, trimmed
12 large mint leaves
30 ml/2 tbsp butter or margarine
5 ml/1 tsp garlic salt
5 ml/1 tsp Worcestershire sauce
5 ml/1 tsp soy sauce
2.5 ml/½ tsp paprika
6 pitta breads, warmed
Lettuce leaves, tomato and cucumber slices

Cut the meat into 2.5 cm/1 in cubes. Thread on to six wooden skewers alternately with the mint leaves. Arrange like the spokes of a wheel in a deep 25 cm/10 in diameter dish. Melt the butter or margarine on Full for 1 minute, then add the garlic salt, Worcestershire sauce, soy sauce and paprika and mix together thoroughly. Brush half the mixture over the kebabs. Cook, uncovered, on Full for 8 minutes, turning the dish twice. Turn the kebabs over and brush with the remaining baste. Cook on Full for a further 8 minutes, turning the dish twice. Allow to stand for 5 minutes. Warm the pitta breads briefly under the grill (broiler) until they puff up, then slice along the long edge to make a pocket. Remove the meat from the skewers and discard the bay leaves. Pack the lamb into the pittas, then add a good helping of the salad to each.

Middle Eastern Lamb with Fruit

Serves 4–6

This delicately spiced and fruited lamb dish is understated elegance, enhanced by its coating of toasted pine nuts and flaked almonds. Serve with yoghurt and buttery rice.

675 g/1½ lb boned lamb, as lean as possible
5 ml/1 tsp ground cinnamon
2.5 ml/½ tsp ground cloves
30 ml/2 tbsp light soft brown sugar
1 onion, chopped
30 ml/2 tbsp lemon juice
10 ml/2 tsp cornflour (cornstarch)
15 ml/1 tbsp cold water
7.5–10 ml/1½–2 tsp salt
400 g/14 oz/1 large can peach slices in natural or apple juice, drained
30 ml/2 tbsp toasted pine nuts
30 ml/2 tbsp flaked (slivered) almonds

Cut the lamb into small cubes. Place in a 1.75 litre/3 pt/7½ cup casserole dish (Dutch oven). Mix together the spices, sugar, onion and lemon juice and add to the dish. Cover with a plate and cook on Full for 5 minutes, then allow to stand for 5 minutes. Repeat three times, stirring well each time. Mix together the cornflour and water to make a smooth paste. Drain the liquid from the lamb and add the cornflour mixture and salt. Pour over the lamb and stir well to mix. Cook, uncovered, on Full for 2 minutes. Stir in the peach slices and cook, uncovered, on Full for a further 1½ minutes. Sprinkle with the pine nuts and almonds and and serve.

Mock Irish Stew

Serves 4

675 g/1½ lb cubed stewing lamb
2 large onions, coarsely grated
450 g/1 lb potatoes, finely diced
300 ml/½ pt/1¼ cups boiling water
5 ml/1 tsp salt
45 ml/3 tbsp chopped parsley

Trim away any excess fat from the lamb. Place the meat and vegetables in a single layer in a deep 25 cm/10 in diameter dish. Cover with clingfilm (plastic wrap) and slit it twice to allow steam to escape. Cook on Full for 15 minutes, turning the dish twice. Mix the water and salt and pour over the meat and vegetables, stirring thoroughly to combine. Cover as before and cook on Full for 20 minutes, turning the dish three times. Allow to stand for 10 minutes. Uncover and sprinkle with the parsley before serving.

Farmer's Wife Lamb Chops

Serves 4

3 cold cooked potatoes, thinly sliced
3 cold cooked carrots, thinly sliced
4 lean lamb chops, 150 g/5 oz each
1 small onion, grated
1 cooking (tart) apple, peeled and grated
30 ml/2 tbsp apple juice
Salt and freshly ground black pepper
15 ml/1 tbsp butter or margarine

Arrange the potato and carrot slices in a single layer over the base of a deep 20 cm/8 in diameter dish. Arrange the chops on top. Sprinkle with the onion and apple and pour the juice over. Season to taste and dot with flakes of the butter or margarine. Cover with clingfilm (plastic wrap) and slit it twice to allow steam to escape. Cook on Full for 15 minutes, turning the dish twice. Allow to stand for 5 minutes before serving.

Lamb Hot-pot

Serves 4

675 g/1½ lb potatoes, very thinly sliced
2 onions, very thinly sliced
3 carrots, very thinly sliced
2 large celery stalks, cut diagonally into thin strips
8 best end of neck lamb chops, about 1 kg/2 lb in all
1 beef stock cube
300 ml/½ pt/1¼ cups boiling water
5 ml/1 tsp salt
25 ml/1½ tbsp melted butter or margarine

Arrange half the prepared vegetables in layers in a lightly greased 2.25 litre/4 pt/10 cup casserole dish (Dutch oven). Place the chops on top and cover with the remaining vegetables. Cover with clingfilm (plastic wrap) and slit it twice to allow steam to escape. Cook on Full for 15 minutes, turning the dish three times. Remove from the microwave and uncover. Crumble the stock cube into the water and add the salt. Pour gently down the side of the casserole. Trickle the butter or margarine over the top. Cover as before and cook on Full for 15 minutes. Allow to stand for 6 minutes before serving.

Lamb Loaf with Mint and Rosemary

Serves 4

450 g/1 lb/4 cups minced (ground) lamb
1 garlic clove, crushed
2.5 ml/½ tsp dried crumbled rosemary
2.5 ml/½ tsp dried mint
30 ml/2 tbsp plain (all-purpose) flour
2 large eggs, beaten
2.5 ml/½ tsp salt
5 ml/1 tsp brown table sauce
Grated nutmeg

Lightly grease a 900 ml/1½ pt/3¾ cup oval pie dish. Mix together all the ingredients except the nutmeg and spread smoothly into the dish. Cover with clingfilm (plastic wrap) and slit it twice to allow steam to escape. Cook on Full for 8 minutes, turning the dish twice. Allow to stand for 4 minutes, then uncover and sprinkle with nutmeg. Cut into portions to serve.

Lamb Bredie with Tomatoes

Serves 6

Prepare as for Chicken Bredie with Tomatoes, but substitute boned and coarsely chopped lamb for the chicken.

Lamb Biriani

Serves 4–6

5 cardamom pods

30 ml/2 tbsp sunflower oil

450 g/1 lb trimmed neck of lamb fillet, cut into small cubes

2 garlic cloves, crushed

20 ml/4 tsp garam masala

225 g/8 oz/1¼ cups easy-cook long-grain rice

600 ml/1 pt/2½ cups hot chicken stock

10 ml/2 tsp salt

125 g/4 oz/1 cup flaked (slivered) almonds, toasted

Split the cardamom pods to remove the seeds, then crush the seeds with a pestle and mortar. Heat the oil in a 1.5 litre/3 pt/7½ cup casserole dish (Dutch oven) on Full for 1½ minutes. Add the lamb, garlic, cardamom seeds and garam masala. Mix well, then arrange round the edge of the dish, leaving a small hollow in the centre. Cover with clingfilm (plastic wrap) and slit it twice to allow steam to escape. Cook on Full for 10 minutes. Uncover and mix in the rice, stock and salt. Cover as before and cook on Full for 15 minutes. Allow to stand for 3 minutes, then spoon out on to warmed plates and sprinkle each portion with the almonds.

Ornate Biriani

Serves 4–6

Prepare as for Lamb Biriani, but arrange the biriani on a warmed serving dish and garnish with chopped hard-boiled (hard-cooked) eggs, tomato wedges, coriander (cilantro) leaves and fried (sautéed) chopped onion.

Moussaka

Serves 6–8

You require a little patience to prepare this multi-layered lamb-based Greek classic but the results are well worth the effort. Poached aubergine (eggplant) slices makes this less rich and easier to digest than some versions.

For the aubergine layers:
675 g/1½ lb aubergines
75 ml/5 tbsp hot water
5 ml/1 tsp salt
15 ml/1 tbsp fresh lemon juice

For the meat layers:
40 g/1½ oz/3 tbsp butter, margarine or olive oil
2 onions, finely chopped
1 garlic clove, crushed
350 g/12 oz/3 cups cold cooked minced (ground) lamb
125 g/4 oz/2 cups fresh white breadcrumbs
Salt and freshly ground black pepper
4 tomatoes, blanched, skinned and sliced

For the sauce:
425 ml/¾ pt/scant 2 cups full- cream milk
40 g/1½ oz/3 tbsp butter or margarine
45 ml/3 tbsp plain (all-purpose) flour

75 g/3 oz/¾ cup Cheddar cheese, grated

1 egg yolk

Moussaka with Potatoes

Serves 6–8

Prepare as for Moussaka, but substitute sliced cooked potatoes for the aubergines (eggplants).

Quick Moussaka

Serves 3–4

A quick alternative with an acceptable flavour and texture.

1 aubergine (eggplant), about 225 g/8 oz
15 ml/1 tbsp cold water
300 ml/½ pt/1¼ cups cold milk
300 ml/½ pt/1¼ cups water
1 packet instant mashed potato to serve 4
225 g/8 oz/2 cups cold cooked minced (ground) lamb
5 ml/1 tsp dried marjoram
5 ml/1 tsp salt
2 garlic cloves, crushed
3 tomatoes, blanched, skinned and sliced
150 ml/¼ pt/2/3 cup thick Greek plain yoghurt
1 egg
Salt and freshly ground black pepper
50 g/2 oz/½ cup Cheddar cheese, grated

Top and tail the aubergine and halve it lengthways. Place in a shallow dish, cut sides uppermost and sprinkle with the cold water. Cover with clingfilm (plastic wrap) and slit it twice to allow steam to escape. Cook on Full for 5½–6 minutes until tender. Allow to stand for 2 minutes, then drain. Pour the milk and water into a bowl and stir in the dried potato. Cover with a plate and cook on Full for 6 minutes. Stir well, then mix in the lamb, marjoram, salt and garlic. Slice the unpeeled aubergine. Arrange alternate layers of aubergine slices and the potato mixture in a 2.25 litre/4 pt/10 cup greased casserole dish (Dutch oven), using half the tomato slices to form a 'sandwich filling' in the centre. Cover with the remaining tomato slices. Beat together the yoghurt and egg and season to taste. Spoon over the tomatoes and sprinkle with the cheese. Cover with clingfilm as before. Cook on Full for 7 minutes. Uncover and brown under a hot grill (broiler) before serving.

Lamb Mince

Serves 4

Prepare as for Basic Mince, but substitute minced (ground) lamb for the minced beef.

Shepherd's Pie

Serves 4

Prepare as for Basic Mince, but substitute lamb mince for beef. Cool to lukewarm, then transfer to a 1 litre/1¾ pt/4½ cup greased pie dish. Top with 750 g/1½ lb hot mashed potato creamed with 15–30 ml/1–2 tbsp butter or margarine and 60 ml/4 tbsp hot milk. Season well with salt and freshly ground black pepper. Spread over the meat mixture, then rough up with a fork. Reheat, uncovered, on Full for 2–3 minutes or brown under a hot grill (broiler).

Country Liver in Red Wine

Serves 4

25 g/1 oz/2 tbsp butter or margarine
2 onions, grated
450 g/1 lb lambs' liver, cut into narrow strips
15 ml/1 tbsp plain (all-purpose) flour
300 ml/½ pt/1¼ cups red wine
15 ml/1 tbsp dark soft brown sugar
1 beef stock cube, crumbled
30 ml/2 tbsp chopped parsley
Salt and freshly ground black pepper
Buttered boiled potatoes and lightly cooked shredded cabbage, to serve

Put the butter or margarine in a deep 25 cm/10 in diameter dish. Melt, uncovered, on Defrost for 2 minutes. Stir in the onions and liver. Cover with a plate and cook on Full for 5 minutes. Mix in all the remaining ingredients except the salt and pepper. Cover with a plate and cook on Full for 6 minutes, stirring twice. Allow to stand for 3 minutes. Season to taste and serve with buttered boiled potatoes and cabbage.

Liver and Bacon

Serves 4–6

2 onions, grated
8 bacon rashers (slices), coarsely chopped
450 g/1 lb lambs' liver, cut into small cubes
45 ml/3 tbsp cornflour (cornstarch)
60 ml/4 tbsp cold water
150 ml/¼ pt/2/3 cup boiling water
Salt and freshly ground black pepper

Put the onions and bacon in a 1.75 litre/3 pt/7½ cup casserole dish (Dutch oven). Cook, uncovered, on Full for 7 minutes, stirring twice. Mix in the liver. Cover with a plate and cook on Full for 8 minutes, stirring three times. Mix the cornflour with the cold water to make a smooth paste. Stir into the liver and onions, then gradually blend in the boiling water. Cover with a plate and cook on Full for 6 minutes, stirring three times. Allow to stand for 4 minutes. Season to taste and serve.

Liver and Bacon with Apple

Serves 4–6

Prepare as for Liver and Bacon, but substitute 1 eating (dessert) apple, peeled and grated, for one of the onions. Substitute apple juice at room temperature for half the boiling water.

Kidneys in Red Wine with Brandy

Serves 4

6 lambs' kidneys
30 ml/2 tbsp butter or margarine
1 onion, finely chopped
30 ml/2 tbsp plain (all-purpose) flour
150 ml/¼ pt/2/3 cup dry red wine
2 beef stock cubes
50 g/2 oz mushrooms, sliced
10 ml/2 tsp tomato purée (paste)
2.5 ml/½ tsp paprika
2.5 ml/½ tsp mustard powder
30 ml/2 tbsp chopped parsley
30 ml/2 tbsp brandy

Skin and halve the kidneys, then cut out and discard the cores with a sharp knife. Slice very thinly. Melt half the butter, uncovered, on Defrost for 1 minute. Stir in the kidneys and set aside. Put the remaining butter and the onion in a 1.5 litre/2½ pt/6 cup dish. Cook, uncovered, on Full for 2 minutes, stirring once. Mix in the flour, then the wine. Cook, uncovered, on Full for 3 minutes, stirring briskly every minute. Crumble in the stock cubes, then stir in the mushrooms, tomato purée, paprika, mustard and the kidneys with the butter or margarine. Mix thoroughly. Cover with clingfilm (plastic wrap) and slit it twice to allow steam to escape. Cook on Full for 5 minutes, turning the dish once. Allow to stand for 3 minutes, then uncover and sprinkle with the parsley. Warm the brandy in a cup on Full for 10–15 seconds. Pour over the kidney mixture and ignite. Serve when the flames have subsided.

Venison Steaks with Oyster Mushrooms and Blue Cheese

Serves 4

Salt and freshly ground black pepper
8 small venison steaks
5 ml/1 tsp juniper berries, crushed
5 ml/1 tsp herbes de Provence
30 ml/2 tbsp olive oil
300 ml/½ pt/1¼ cups dry red wine
60 ml/4 tbsp rich beef stock
60 ml/4 tbsp gin
1 onion, chopped
225 g/8 oz oyster mushrooms, trimmed and sliced
250 ml/8 fl oz/1 cup single (light) cream
30 ml/2 tbsp redcurrant jelly (clear conserve)
60 ml/4 tbsp blue cheese, crumbled
30 ml/2 tbsp chopped parsley

Season the venison to taste, then work in the juniper berries and herbes de Provence. Heat the oil in a browning dish on Full for 2 minutes. Add the steaks and cook, uncovered, on Full for 3 minutes, turning once. Add the wine, stock, gin, onion, mushrooms, cream and redcurrant jelly. Cover with clingfilm (plastic wrap) and slit it twice to allow steam to escape. Cook on Medium for 25 minutes, turning the dish four times. Mix in the cheese. Cover with a heatproof plate and cook on Full for 2 minutes. Allow to stand for 3 minutes, then uncover and serve garnished with the parsley.

Cooking Small Pasta

Follow the directions for cooking large pasta but cook for only 4–5 minutes. Cover and stand for 3 minutes, then drain and serve.

Chinese Noodle and Mushroom Salad with Walnuts

Serves 6

30 ml/2 tbsp sesame oil
175 g/6 oz mushrooms, sliced
250 g/9 oz thread egg noodles
7.5 ml/1½ tsp salt
75 g/3 oz/¾ cup chopped walnuts
5 spring onions (scallions), chopped
30 ml/2 tbsp soy sauce

Heat the oil, uncovered, on Defrost for 2½ minutes. Add the mushrooms. Cover with a plate and cook on Full for 3 minutes, stirring twice. Set aside. Put the noodles in a large bowl and add enough boiling water to come 5 cm/2 in above the level of the pasta. Stir in the salt. Cook, uncovered, on Full for 4–5 minutes until the noodles swell and are just tender. Drain and allow to cool. Mix in the remaining ingredients including the mushrooms and toss well to mix.

Pepper Macaroni

Serves 2

300 ml/½ pt/1¼ cups tomato juice
125 g/4 oz/1 cup elbow macaroni
5 ml/1 tsp salt
30 ml/2 tbsp white wine, heated
1 small red or green (bell) pepper, seeded and chopped
45 ml/3 tbsp olive oil
75 g/3 oz/¾ cup Gruyère (Swiss) or Emmental cheese, grated
30 ml/2 tbsp chopped parsley

Pour the tomato juice into a 1.25 litre/2¼ pt/5½ cup dish. Cover with a plate and heat on Full for 3½–4 minutes until very hot and bubbling. Stir in all the remaining ingredients except the cheese and parsley. Cover as before and cook on Full for 10 minutes, stirring twice. Allow to stand for 5 minutes. Sprinkle with the cheese and parsley. Reheat, uncovered, on Full for about 1 minute until the cheese melts.

Family Macaroni Cheese

Serves 6–7

For convenience, this recipe is for a large family-sized meal, but any leftovers can be reheated in portions in the microwave.

350 g/12 oz/3 cups elbow macaroni
10 ml/2 tsp salt
30 ml/2 tbsp cornflour (cornstarch)
600 ml/1 pt/2½ cups cold milk
1 egg, beaten
10 ml/2 tsp made mustard
Freshly ground black pepper
275 g/10 oz/2½ cups Cheddar cheese, grated

Put the macaroni in a deep dish. Stir in the salt and sufficient boiling water to come 5 cm/2 in above the level of the pasta. Cook, uncovered, on Full for about 10 minutes until just tender, stirring three times. Drain if necessary, then leave to stand while preparing the sauce. In a separate large bowl, mix the cornflour smoothly with some of the cold milk, then mix in the remainder. Cook, uncovered, on Full for 6–7 minutes until smoothly thickened, whisking every minute. Mix in the egg, mustard and pepper followed by two-thirds of the cheese and all the macaroni. Mix thoroughly with a fork. Spread evenly into a buttered 30 cm/12 in diameter dish. Sprinkle the remaining cheese over the top. Reheat, uncovered, on Full for 4–5 minutes. If liked, brown quickly under a hot grill (broiler) before serving.

Classic Macaroni Cheese

Serves 4–5

This version is slightly richer than Family Macaroni Cheese and lends itself to a number of variations.

225 g/8 oz/2 cups elbow macaroni
7.5 ml/1½ tsp salt
30 ml/2 tbsp butter or margarine
30 ml/2 tbsp plain (all-purpose) flour
300 ml/½ pt/1¼ cups milk
225 g/8 oz/2 cups Cheddar cheese, grated
5–10 ml/1–2 tsp made mustard
Salt and freshly ground black pepper

Put the macaroni in a deep dish. Stir in the salt and sufficient boiling water to come 5 cm/2 in above the level of the pasta. Cook, uncovered, on Full for 8–10 minutes until just tender, stirring two or three times. Stand for 3–4 minutes inside the microwave. Drain if necessary, then leave to stand while preparing the sauce. Melt the butter or margarine, uncovered, on Defrost for 1–1½ minutes. Stir in the flour, then gradually blend in the milk. Cook, uncovered, on Full for 6–7 minutes until smoothly thickened, whisking every minute. Mix in two-thirds of the cheese, followed by the mustard and seasoning, then the macaroni. Spread evenly in a 20 cm/8 in diameter dish. Sprinkle with the remaining cheese. Reheat, uncovered, on Full for 3–4 minutes. If liked, brown quickly under a hot grill (broiler) before serving.

Macaroni Cheese with Stilton

Serves 4–5

Prepare as for Classic Macaroni Cheese, but substitute 100 g/3½ oz/1 cup crumbled Stilton for half the Cheddar cheese.

Macaroni Cheese with Bacon

Serves 4–5

Prepare as for Classic Macaroni Cheese, but stir in 6 rashers (slices) streaky bacon, grilled (broiled) until crisp then crumbled, with the mustard and seasoning.

Macaroni Cheese with Tomatoes

Serves 4–5

Prepare as for Classic Macaroni Cheese, but place a layer of tomato slices from about 3 skinned tomatoes on top of the pasta before sprinkling with the remaining cheese.

Spaghetti Carbonara

Serves 4

75 ml/5 tbsp double (heavy) cream
2 large eggs
100 g/4 oz/1 cup Parma ham, chopped
175 g/6 oz/1½ cups grated Parmesan cheese
350 g/12 oz spaghetti or other large pasta

Beat together the cream and eggs. Stir in the ham and 90 ml/6 tbsp of the Parmesan. Cook the spaghetti as directed. Drain and place in a serving dish. Add the cream mixture and toss all together with two wooden forks or spoons. Cover with kitchen paper and reheat on Full for 1½ minutes. Serve each portion topped with the remaining Parmesan.

Pizza-style Macaroni Cheese

Serves 4–5

225 g/8 oz/2 cups elbow macaroni
7.5 ml/1½ tsp salt
30 ml/2 tbsp butter or margarine
30 ml/2 tbsp plain (all-purpose) flour
300 ml/½ pt/1¼ cups milk
125 g/4 oz/1 cup Cheddar cheese, grated
125 g/4 oz/1 cup Mozzarella cheese, grated
5–10 ml/1–2 tsp made mustard
Salt and freshly ground black pepper
212 g/7 oz/1 small can tuna in oil, drained and oil reserved
12 stoned (pitted) black olives, sliced
1 canned pimiento, sliced
2 tomatoes, blanched, skinned and coarsely chopped
5–10 ml/1–2 tsp red or green pesto (optional)
Basil leaves, to garnish

Put the macaroni in a deep dish. Stir in the salt and sufficient boiling water to come 5 cm/2 in above the level of the pasta. Cook, uncovered, on Full for 8–10 minutes until just tender, stirring two or three times. Stand for 3–4 minutes inside the microwave. Drain if necessary, then leave to stand while preparing the sauce. Melt the butter or margarine, uncovered, on Defrost for 1–1½ minutes. Stir in the flour, then gradually blend in the milk. Cook, uncovered, on Full for 6–7 minutes until smoothly thickened, whisking every minute. Mix in two-thirds of each cheese, followed by the mustard and seasoning. Stir in the macaroni, tuna, 15 ml/1 tbsp of the tuna oil, the olives, pimiento, tomatoes and pesto, if using. Spread evenly in a 20 cm/8 in diameter dish. Sprinkle with the remaining cheeses. Reheat, uncovered, on Full for 3–4 minutes. If liked, brown quickly under a hot grill (broiler) before serving garnished with basil leaves.

Spaghetti Cream with Spring Onions

Serves 4

150 ml/¼ pt/2/3 cup double (heavy) cream
1 egg yolk
150 g/5 oz/1¼ cups grated Parmesan cheese
8 spring onions (scallions), finely chopped
Salt and freshly ground black pepper
350 g/12 oz spaghetti or other large pasta

Beat together the cream, egg yolk, 45 ml/3 tbsp of the Parmesan and the spring onions. Season well to taste. Cook the spaghetti as directed. Drain and place in a serving dish. Add the cream mixture and toss all together with two wooden forks or spoons. Cover with kitchen paper and reheat on Full for 1½ minutes. Offer the remaining Parmesan cheese separately.

Spaghetti Bolognese

Serves 4–6

450 g/1 lb/4 cups lean minced (ground) beef
1 garlic clove, crushed
1 large onion, grated
1 green (bell) pepper, seeded and finely chopped
5 ml/1 tsp Italian seasoning or dried mixed herbs
400 g/14 oz/1 large can chopped tomatoes
45 ml/3 tbsp tomato purée (paste)
1 beef stock cube
75 ml/5 tbsp red wine or water
15 ml/1 tbsp dark soft brown sugar
5 ml/1 tsp salt
Freshly ground black pepper
350 g/12 oz freshly cooked and drained spaghetti or other pasta
Grated Parmesan cheese

Combine the beef with the garlic in a 1.75 litre/3 pt/7½ cup dish. Cook, uncovered, on Full for 5 minutes. Mix in all the remaining ingredients except the salt, pepper and spaghetti. Cover with a plate and cook on Full for 15 minutes, stirring four times with a fork to break up the meat. Allow to stand for 4 minutes. Season with the salt and pepper to taste and serve with the spaghetti. Offer the Parmesan cheese separately.

Spaghetti with Turkey Bolognese Sauce

Serves 4

Prepare as for Spaghetti Bolognese, but substitute minced (ground) turkey for the beef.

Spaghetti with Ragu Sauce

Serves 4

A traditional and economical sauce, first used in England in Soho trattorias shortly after World War Two.

20 ml/4 tsp olive oil
1 large onion, finely chopped
1 garlic clove, crushed
1 small carrot, grated
250 g/8 oz/2 cups lean minced (ground) beef
10 ml/2 tsp plain (all-purpose) flour
15 ml/1 tbsp tomato purée (paste)
300 m/½ pt/1¼ cups beef stock
45 ml/3 tbsp dry white wine
1.5 ml/¼ tsp dried basil
1 small bay leaf
175 g/6 oz mushrooms, coarsely chopped
Salt and freshly ground black pepper
350 g/12 oz freshly cooked and drained spaghetti or other pasta
Grated Parmesan cheese

Place the oil, onion, garlic and carrot in a 1.75 litre/3 pt/7½ cup dish. Heat, uncovered, on Full for 6 minutes. Add all the remaining ingredients except the salt, pepper and spaghetti. Cover with a plate and cook on Full for 11 minutes, stirring three times. Allow to stand for 4 minutes. Season with salt and pepper, remove the bay leaf and serve with the spaghetti. Offer the Parmesan cheese separately.

Spaghetti with Butter

Serves 4

350 g/12 oz pasta
60 ml/4 tbsp butter or olive oil
Grated Parmesan cheese

Cook the pasta as directed. Drain and place in a large dish with the butter or olive oil. Toss with two spoons until the pasta is well coated. Spoon on to four warmed plates and heap grated Parmesan cheese on each.

Pasta with Garlic

Serves 4

350 g/12 oz pasta
2 cloves garlic, crushed
50 g/2 oz butter
10 ml/2 tsp olive oil
30 ml/2 tbsp chopped parsley
Grated Parmesan cheese
Rocket or radicchio leaves, shredded

Cook the pasta as directed. Heat the garlic, butter and oil on Full for 1½ minutes. Stir in the parsley. Drain the pasta and place in a serving dish. Add the garlic mixture and toss all together with two wooden spoons. Serve straight away sprinkled with Parmesan and garnished with shredded rocket or radicchio leaves.

Spaghetti with Beef and Mixed Vegetable Bolognese Sauce

Serves 4

30 ml/2 tbsp olive oil
1 large onion, finely chopped
2 garlic cloves, crushed
4 rashers (slices) streaky bacon, chopped
1 celery stalk, chopped
1 carrot, grated
125 g/4 oz button mushrooms, thinly sliced
225 g/8 oz/2 cups lean minced (ground) beef
30 ml/2 tbsp plain (all-purpose) flour
1 wine glass dry red wine
150 ml/¼ pt/2/3 cup passata (sieved tomatoes)
60 ml/4 tbsp beef stock
2 large tomatoes, blanched, skinned and chopped
15 ml/1 tbsp dark soft brown sugar
1.5 ml/¼ tsp grated nutmeg
15 ml/1 tbsp chopped basil leaves
Salt and freshly ground black pepper
350 g/12 oz freshly cooked and drained spaghetti
Grated Parmesan cheese

Put the oil, onion, garlic, bacon, celery and carrot in a 2 litre/3½ pt/8½ cup dish. Add the mushrooms and meat. Cook, uncovered, on Full for 6 minutes, stirring twice with a fork to break up the meat. Mix in all the remaining ingredients except the salt, pepper and spaghetti. Cover with a plate and cook on Full for 13–15 minutes, stirring three times. Allow to stand for 4 minutes. Season with salt and pepper and serve with the pasta. Offer the Parmesan cheese separately.

Spaghetti with Meat Sauce and Cream

Serves 4

Prepare as for Spaghetti with Beef and Mixed Vegetable Bolognese Sauce, but stir in 30–45 ml/2–3 tbsp double (heavy) cream at the end.

Spaghetti with Marsala Meat Sauce

Serves 4

Prepare as for Spaghetti with Beef and Mixed Vegetable Bolognese Sauce, but substitute marsala for the wine and add 45 ml/3 tbsp Marscapone cheese at the end.

Pasta alla Marinara

Serves 4

This means 'sailor style' and comes from Naples.
30 ml/2 tbsp olive oil
3–4 garlic cloves, crushed
8 large tomatoes, blanched, skinned and chopped
5 ml/1 tsp finely chopped mint
15 ml/1 tbsp finely chopped basil leaves
Salt and freshly ground black pepper
350 g/12 oz freshly cooked and drained pasta
Grated Pecorino or Parmesan cheese, to serve

Put all the ingredients except the pasta in a 1.25 litre/2¼ pt/5½ cup dish. Cover with a plate and cook on Full for 6–7 minutes, stirring three times. Serve with the pasta and offer the Pecorino or Parmesan cheese separately.

Pasta Matriciana

Serves 4

A rustic pasta sauce from the central Abruzzo region in Italy.

30 ml/2 tbsp olive oil
1 onion, chopped
5 rashers (slices) unsmoked streaky bacon, coarsely chopped
8 tomatoes, blanched, skinned and chopped
2–3 garlic cloves, crushed
350 g/12 oz freshly cooked and drained pasta
Grated Pecorino or Parmesan cheese, to serve

Put all the ingredients except the pasta in a 1.25 litre/2¼ pt/5½ cup dish. Cover with a plate and cook on Full for 6 minutes, stirring twice. Serve with the pasta and offer the Pecorino or Parmesan cheese separately.

Pasta with Tuna and Capers

Serves 4

15 ml/1 tbsp butter
200 g/7 oz/1 small can tuna in oil
60 ml/4 tbsp vegetable stock or white wine
15 ml/1 tbsp capers, chopped
30 ml/2 tbsp chopped parsley
350 g/12 oz freshly cooked and drained pasta
Grated Parmesan cheese

Put the butter in a 600 ml/1 pt/2½ cup dish and melt, uncovered, on Defrost for 1½ minutes. Add the contents of the can of tuna and flake the fish. Stir in the stock or wine, capers and parsley. Cover with a plate and heat on Full for 3–4 minutes. Serve with the pasta and offer the Parmesan cheese separately.

Pasta Napoletana

Serves 4

This flamboyant tomato sauce from Naples, with a warm and colourful flavour, is best made in summer when tomatoes are at their most abundant.

8 large ripe tomatoes, blanched, skinned and coarsely chopped
30 ml/2 tbsp olive oil
1 onion, chopped
2–4 garlic cloves, crushed
1 celery stalk, finely chopped
15 ml/1 tbsp chopped basil leaves
10 ml/2 tsp light soft brown sugar
60 ml/4 tbsp water or red wine
Salt and freshly ground black pepper
30 ml/2 tbsp chopped parsley
350 g/12 oz freshly cooked and drained pasta
Grated Parmesan cheese

Put the tomatoes, oil, onion, garlic, celery, basil, sugar and water or wine in a 1.25 litre/2¼ pt/5½ cup dish. Mix well. Cover with a plate and cook on Full for 7 minutes, stirring twice. Season to taste, then stir in the parsley. Serve straight away with the pasta and offer the Parmesan cheese separately.

Pasta Pizzaiola

Serves 4

Prepare as for Pasta Napoletana, but increase the tomatoes to 10, omit the onion, celery and water and use double the amount of parsley. Add 15 ml/1 tbsp fresh or 2.5 ml/½ tsp dried oregano with the parsley.

Pasta with Peas

Serves 4

Prepare as for Pasta Napoletana, but add 125 g/4 oz/1 cup coarsely chopped ham and 175 g/6 oz/1½ cups fresh peas to the tomatoes with the other ingredients. Cook for 9–10 minutes.

Pasta with Chicken Liver Sauce

Serves 4

225 g/8 oz chicken livers
30 ml/2 tbsp plain (all-purpose) flour
15 ml/1 tbsp butter
15 ml/1 tbsp olive oil
1–2 garlic cloves, crushed
125 g/4 oz mushrooms, sliced
150 ml/¼ pt/⅔ cup hot water
150 ml/¼ pt/⅔ cup dry red wine
Salt and freshly ground black pepper
350 g/12 oz pasta, freshly cooked and drained

Pasta with Anchovies

Serves 4

30 ml/2 tbsp olive oil
15 ml/1 tbsp butter
2 garlic cloves, crushed
50 g/2 oz/1 small can anchovy fillets in oil
45 ml/3 tbsp chopped parsley
2.5 ml/½ tsp dried basil
Freshly ground black pepper
350 g/12 oz freshly cooked and drained pasta

Put the oil, butter and garlic in a 600 ml/1 pt/2½ cup dish. Chop the anchovies and add with the oil from the can. Mix in the parsley, basil and pepper to taste. Cover with a plate and cook on Full for 3–3½ minutes. Serve straight away with the pasta.

Ravioli with Sauce

Serves 4

350 g/12 oz/3 cups ravioli

Cook as for large pasta, then serve with any of the tomato-based pasta sauces above.

Tortellini

Serves 4

Allow about 250 g/9 oz bought tortellini and cook as for large fresh or dried pasta. Drain thoroughly, add 25 g/1 oz/2 tbsp unsalted (sweet) butter and toss thoroughly. Serve each portion dusted with grated Parmesan cheese.

Lasagne

Serves 4–6

45 ml/3 tbsp hot water
Spaghetti Bolognese sauce
9–10 sheets no-need-to-precook plain, green (verdi) or brown (wholewheat) lasagne
Cheese Sauce
25 g/1 oz/¼ cup grated Parmesan cheese
30 ml/2 tbsp butter
Grated nutmeg

Oil or butter a 20 cm/8 in square dish. Add the hot water to the Bolognese sauce. Place a layer of lasagne sheets in the bottom of the dish, then a layer of Bolognese sauce, then a layer of cheese sauce. Continue with the layers, finishing with the cheese sauce. Sprinkle with the Parmesan cheese, dot with the butter and dust with nutmeg. Cook, uncovered, for 15 minutes, turning the dish twice. Allow to stand for 5 minutes, then continue to cook for a further 15 minutes or until the lasagne feels soft when a knife is pushed through the centre. (The cooking time will vary depending on the initial temperature of the two sauces.)

Pizza Napoletana

Makes 4

The microwave does a great job on pizzas, reminiscent of the ones you can find all over Italy and in Naples in particular.

30 ml/2 tbsp olive oil
2 onions, peeled and finely chopped
1 garlic clove, crushed
150 g/5 oz/2/3 cup tomato purée (paste)
Basic White or Brown Bread Dough
350 g/12 oz/3 cups Mozzarella cheese, grated
10 ml/2 tsp dried oregano
50 g/2 oz/1 small can anchovy fillets in oil

Cook the oil, onions and garlic, uncovered, on Full for 5 minutes, stirring twice. Mix in the tomato purée and set aside. Divide the dough equally into four pieces. Roll each into a round large enough to cover an oiled and floured 20 cm/8 in flat plate. Cover with kitchen paper and leave to stand for 30 minutes. Spread each with the tomato mixture. Mix the cheese with the oregano and sprinkle equally over each pizza. Garnish with the anchovies. Bake individually, covered with kitchen paper, on Full for 5 minutes, turning twice. Eat straight away.

Pizza Margherita

Makes 4

Prepare as for Pizza Napoletana, but substitute dried basil for the oregano and omit the anchovies.

Seafood Pizza

Makes 4

Prepare as for Pizza Napoletana. When cooked, stud with prawns (shrimp), mussels, clams etc.

Pizza Siciliana

Makes 4

Prepare as for Pizza Napoletana. When cooked, stud with 18 small black olives between the anchovies.

Mushroom Pizza

Makes 4

Prepare as for Pizza Napoletana, but sprinkle 100 g/3½ oz thinly sliced mushrooms over the tomato mixture before adding the cheese and herbs. Cook for an extra 30 seconds.

Ham and Pineapple Pizza

Makes 4

Prepare as for Pizza Napoletana, but sprinkle 125 g/4 oz/1 cup chopped ham over the tomato mixture before adding the cheese and herbs. Chop 2 canned pineapple rings and scatter over the top of the pizza. Cook for an extra 45 seconds.

Pepperoni Pizzas

Makes 4

Prepare as for Pizza Napoletana, but top each pizza with 6 thin slices of pepperoni sausage.

Buttered Flaked Almonds

A splendid topping for sweet and savoury dishes.

15 ml/1 tbsp unsalted (sweet) butter
50 g/2 oz/½ cup flaked (slivered) almonds
Plain or flavoured salt or caster (superfine) sugar

Put the butter in a shallow 20 cm/8 in diameter dish. Melt, uncovered, on Full for 45–60 seconds. Add the almonds and cook, uncovered, on Full for 5–6 minutes until golden brown, stirring and turning every minute. Sprinkle with salt for topping savoury dishes, caster sugar for sweet.

Flaked Almonds in Garlic Butter

Prepare as for Buttered Flaked Almonds, but use bought garlic butter. This makes a smart topping for dishes like mashed potato and can also be added to creamy soups.

Dried Chestnuts

The microwave enables dried chestnuts to be cooked and usable in under 2 hours without soaking overnight followed by prolonged cooking. Also the hard job of peeling has already been done for you.

Wash 250 g/8 oz/2 cups dried chestnuts. Put into a 1.75 litre/3 pt/7½ cup dish. Stir in 600 ml/1 pt/2½ cups boiling water. Cover with a plate and cook on Full for 15 minutes, turning the dish three times. Stand in the microwave for 15 minutes. Repeat with the same cooking and standing times. Uncover, add a further 150 ml/¼ pt/2/3 cup boiling water and stir round. Cover as before and cook on Full for 10 minutes, stirring twice. Allow to stand for 15 minutes before using.

Drying Herbs

If you grow your own herbs but find it difficult to dry them in a damp and unpredictable climate, the microwave will do the job for you effectively, efficiently and cleanly in next to no time, so your annual crop can be savoured through the winter months. Each variety of herb should be dried by itself to keep the flavour intact. If you want to later on, you can make up your own blends by mixing several dried herbs together.

Start by cutting the herbs off their shrubs with secateurs or scissors. Pull the leaves (needles in the case of rosemary) off the stalks and pack them loosely into a 300 ml/½ pt/1¼ cup measuring jug, filling it almost to overflowing. Tip into a colander (strainer) and rinse them quickly and gently under cold running water. Drain thoroughly, then dry between the folds of a clean, dry tea towel (dish cloth). Put on top of a double thickness of kitchen paper placed directly on the microwave turntable. Heat, uncovered, on Full for 5–6 minutes, carefully moving the herbs about on the paper two or three times. As soon as they sound like autumn leaves rustling and have lost their bright green colour, you can assume the herbs are dried through. If not, continue to heat for 1–1½ minutes. Remove from the oven and allow to cool. Crush the dried herbs by rubbing them between your hands.

Transfer to airtight jars with stoppers and label. Store away from bright light.

Crisping Breadcrumbs

High-quality pale breadcrumbs – as opposed to marigold-yellow packet ones – are made perfectly in the microwave and turn crisp and brittle without browning. The bread can be fresh or stale but fresh will take a little longer to dry. Crumble 3½ large slices of white or brown bread with crusts into fine crumbs. Spread the crumbs into a shallow 25 cm/10 in diameter dish. Cook, uncovered, on Full for 5–6 minutes, stirring four times, until you can feel in your fingers that the crumbs are dry and crisp. Allow to cool, stirring round from time to time, then store in an airtight container. They will keep almost indefinitely in a cool place.

Nut Burgers

Makes 12

These are by no means new, particularly to vegetarians and vegans, but the combination of nuts gives these burgers an outstanding flavour, and the crunchy texture is equally appetising. They can be served hot with a sauce, cold with salad and mayonnaise, halved horizontally and used as a sandwich filling, or eaten just as they are for a snack.

30 ml/2 tbsp butter or margarine
125 g/4 oz/1 cup unskinned whole almonds
125 g/4 oz/1 cup pecan nut pieces
125 g/4 oz/1 cup cashew nut pieces, toasted
125 g/4 oz/2 cups fresh soft brown breadcrumbs
1 medium onion, grated
2.5 ml/½ tsp salt
5 ml/1 tsp made mustard
30 ml/2 tbsp cold milk

Melt the butter or margarine, uncovered, on Full for 1–1½ minutes. Grind the nuts fairly finely in a blender or food processor. Tip out and combine with the remaining ingredients including the butter or margarine. Divide into 12 equal pieces and shape into ovals. Arrange round the edge of a large greased plate. Cook, uncovered, on Full for 4 minutes, turning once. Allow to stand for 2 minutes.

Nutkin Cake

Serves 6–8

Prepare as for Nut Burgers, but substitute 350 g/12 oz/3 cups ground mixed nuts of your choice for the almonds, pecans and cashews. Shape into a 20 cm/8 in round and put on a greased plate. Cook, uncovered, on Full for 3 minutes. Allow to stand for 5 minutes, then cook on Full for a further 2½ minutes. Allow to stand for 2 minutes. Serve hot or cold, cut into wedges.

Buckwheat

Serves 4

Also known as Saracen corn and native to Russia, buckwheat is related to no other grain. It is the small fruit of a sweetly perfumed pink-flowering plant which is a member of the dock family. The basis of blinis (or Russian pancakes), the grain is a hearty, earthy staple and is a healthy substitute for potatoes with meat and poultry.

175 g/6 oz/1 cup buckwheat
1 egg, beaten
5 ml/1 tsp salt
750 ml/1¼ pts/3 cups boiling water

Mix the buckwheat and egg in a 2 litre/3½ pt/8½ cup dish. Toast, uncovered, on Full for 4 minutes, stirring and breaking up with a fork every minute. Add the salt and water. Stand on a plate in the microwave in case of spillage and cook, uncovered, on Full for 22 minutes, stirring four times. Cover with a plate and allow to stand for 4 minutes. Fork round before serving.

Bulgar

Serves 6–8

Also called burghal, burghul or cracked wheat, this grain is one of the staples of the Middle East. It is now widely available from supermarkets and health food shops.

225 g/8 oz/1¼ cups bulgar
600 ml/1 pt/2½ cups boiling water
5–7.5 ml/1–1½ tsp salt

Put the bulgar in a 1.75 litre/3 pt/7½ cup dish. Toast, uncovered, on Full for 3 minutes, stirring every minute. Stir in the boiling water and salt. Cover with a plate and allow to stand for 6–15 minutes, depending on the variety of bulgar used, until the grain is al dente, like pasta. Fluff up with a fork and eat hot or cold.

Bulgar with Fried Onion

Serves 4

1 onion, grated
15 ml/1 tbsp olive or sunflower
1 quantity Bulgar

Put the onion and oil in a small dish. Cook, uncovered, on Full for 4 minutes, stirring three times. Add to the cooked bulgar at the same time as the water and salt.

Tabbouleh

Serves 4

Coloured deep green by the parsley, this dish evokes the Lebanon and is one of the most appetising salads imaginable, a perfect accompaniment to many dishes from vegetarian nut cutlets to roast lamb. It also makes an attractive starter, arranged over salad greens on individual plates.

1 quantity Bulgar
120–150 ml/4–5 fl oz/½–2/3 cup finely chopped flatleaf parsley
30 ml/2 tbsp chopped mint leaves
1 medium onion, finely grated
15 ml/1 tbsp olive oil
Salt and freshly ground black pepper
Salad leaves
Diced tomatoes, diced cucumber and black olives, to garnish

Cook the bulgar as directed. Transfer half the quantity to a bowl and mix in the parsley, mint, onion, oil and plenty of salt and pepper to taste. When cold, arrange on salad leaves and decorate attractively with the garnish. Use the remaining bulgar in any way you wish.

Sultan's Salad

Serves 4

A personal favourite and, topped with pieces of Feta cheese and served with pitta bread, it makes a complete meal.

1 quantity Bulgar
1–2 garlic cloves, crushed
1 carrot, grated
15 ml/1 tbsp chopped mint leaves
60 ml/4 tbsp chopped parsley
Juice of 1 large lemon, strained
45 ml/3 tbsp olive or sunflower oil, or a mixture of both
Salad greens
Toasted almonds and green olives, to garnish

Cook the bulgar as directed, then stir in the garlic, carrot, mint, parsley, lemon juice and oil. Arrange on a plate lined with salad greens and stud with toasted almonds and green olives.

Couscous

Serves 4

Couscous is both a grain and the name of a North African meat or vegetable stew. Made from durum wheat semolina (cream of wheat), it looks like tiny, perfectly rounded pearls. It used to be hand-made by dedicated and talented home cooks but is now available in packets and can be cooked in a flash, thanks to a French technique that does away with the laborious and slow task of steaming. You can substitute couscous for any of the dishes made with bulgar (pages 209–10).

250 g/9 oz/1½ cups bought couscous
300 ml/½ pt/1¼ cups boiling water
5–10 ml/1–2 tsp salt

Put the couscous in a 1.75 litre/3 pt/7½ cup dish and toast, uncovered, on Full for 3 minutes, stirring every minute. Add the water and salt and fork round. Cover with a plate and cook on Full for 1 minute. Allow to stand in the microwave for 5 minutes. Fluff up with a fork before serving.

Grits

Serves 4

Grits (hominy grits) is a an almost-white North American cereal based on maize (corn). It is eaten with hot milk and sugar or with butter and salt and pepper. It is available from speciality food shops like Harrods in London.

150 g/5 oz/scant 1 cup grits
150 ml/¼ pt/2/3 cup cold water
600 ml/1 pt/2½ cups boiling water
5 ml/1 tsp salt

Put the grits in a 2.5 litre/4½ pt/11 cup bowl. Mix smoothly with the cold water, then stir in the boiling water and salt. Cook, uncovered, on Full for 8 minutes, stirring four times. Cover with a plate and allow to stand for 3 minutes before serving.

Gnocchi alla Romana

Serves 4

Gnocchi is often to be found in Italian restaurants, where it is well liked. It makes a substantial and wholesome lunch or supper dish with salad and uses economical ingredients.

600 ml/1 pt/2½ cups cold milk
150 g/5 oz/¾ cup semolina (cream of wheat)
5 ml/1 tsp salt
50 g/2 oz/¼ cup butter or margarine
75 g/3 oz/¾ cup grated Parmesan cheese
2.5 ml/½ tsp continental made mustard
1.5 ml/¼ tsp grated nutmeg
1 large egg, beaten
Mixed salad
Tomato ketchup (catsup)

Mix half the cold milk smoothly with the semolina in a 1.5 litre/2½ pt/6 cup dish. Heat the remaining milk, uncovered, on Full for 3 minutes. Stir into the semolina with the salt. Cook, uncovered, on Full for 7 minutes until very thick, stirring four or five times to keep the mixture smooth. Remove from the microwave and mix in half the butter, half the cheese and all the mustard, nutmeg and egg. Cook, uncovered, on Full for 1 minute. Cover with a plate and allow to stand for 1 minute. Spread in an oiled or buttered shallow 23 cm/9 in square dish. Cover loosely with kitchen paper and leave in the cool until firm and set. Cut into 2.5 cm/1 in squares. Arrange in a 23 cm/9 in buttered round dish in overlapping rings. Sprinkle with the remaining cheese, dot with flakes of the remaining butter and reheat in a hot oven for 15 minutes until golden brown. Serve very hot with salad and tomato sauce.

Ham Gnocchi

Serves 4

Prepare as for Gnocchi alla Romana, but add 75 g/3 oz/¾ cup chopped Parma ham with the warm milk.

Millet

Serves 4–6

A pleasing and delicate grain, related to sorghum, which is an off-beat substitute for rice. If eaten with pulses (peas, beans and lentils), it makes a well-balanced, protein-rich meal.

175 g/6 oz/1 cup millet
750 ml/1¼ pts/3 cups boiling water or stock
5 ml/1 tsp salt

Put the millet in a 2 litre/3½ pt/8½ cup dish. Toast, uncovered, on Full for 4 minutes, stirring twice. Mix in the water and salt. Stand on a plate in case of spillage. Cook, uncovered, on Full for 20–25 minutes until all the water has been absorbed. Fluff up with a fork and eat straight away.

Polenta

Serves 6

A bright yellow grain made from corn, similar to semolina (cream of wheat) but coarser. It is a staple starch food in Italy and Romania, where it is much respected and often eaten as a side dish with meat, poultry, egg and vegetable dishes. In recent years it has become a trendy restaurant speciality, often cut into squares and served grilled (broiled) or fried (sautéed) with the sauces similar to those used for spaghetti.

150 g/5 oz/¾ cup polenta
5 ml/1 tsp salt
125 ml/¼ pt/2/3 cup cold water
600 ml/1 pt/2½ cups boiling water or stock

Put the polenta and salt in a 2 litre/3½ pt/8½ cup dish. Blend smoothly with the cold water. Gradually mix in the boiling water or stock. Stand on a plate in case of spillage. Cook, uncovered, on Full for 7–8 minutes until very thick, stirring four times. Cover with a plate and allow to stand for 3 minutes before serving.

Grilled Polenta

Serves 6

Prepare as for Polenta. When cooked, spread in a buttered or oiled 23 cm/9 in square dish. Smooth the top with a knife dipped in and out of hot water. Cover loosely with kitchen paper and allow to cool completely. Cut into squares, brush with olive or corn oil and grill (broil) or fry (sauté) conventionally until golden brown.

Polenta with Pesto

Serves 6

Prepare as for Polenta, but add 20 ml/4 tsp red or green pesto with the boiling water.

Polenta with Sun-dried Tomato or Olive Paste

Serves 6

Prepare as for Polenta, but add 45 ml/3 tbsp sun-dried tomato or olive paste with the boiling water.

Quinoa

Serves 2–3

A fairly new-on-the-scene high-protein grain from Peru with a curiously crunchy texture and slightly smoky flavour. It goes with all foods and makes a novel substitute for rice.

125 g/4 oz/2/3 cup quinoa
2.5 ml/½ tsp salt
550 ml/18 fl oz/2 1/3 cups boiling water

Put the quinoa in a 1.75 litre/3 pt/7½ cup bowl. Toast, uncovered, on Full for 3 minutes, stirring once. Add the salt and water and mix in thoroughly. Cook on Full for 15 minutes, stirring four times. Cover and allow to stand for 2 minutes.

Romanian Polenta

Serves 4

Romania's notoriously rich national dish – mamaliga.

1 quantity Polenta
75 g/3 oz/1/3 cup butter
4 freshly poached large eggs
100 g/4 oz/1 cup Feta cheese, crumbled
150 ml/¼ pt/2/3 cup soured (dairy sour) cream

Prepare the polenta and leave in the dish in which it was cooked. Beat in half the butter. Spoon equal mounds on to four warmed plates and make an indentation in each. Fill with the eggs, sprinkle with the cheese and top with the remaining butter and the cream. Eat straight away.

Curried Rice

Serves 4

Suitable as an accompaniment for most oriental and Asiatic foods, especially Indian.

30 ml/2 tbsp groundnut (peanut) oil
2 onions, finely chopped
225 g/8 oz/1 cup basmati rice
2 small bay leaves
2 whole cloves
Seeds from 4 cardamom pods
30–45 ml/2–3 tbsp mild curry powder
5 ml/1 tsp salt
600 ml/1 pt/2½ cups boiling water or vegetable stock

Put the oil in a 2.25 litre/4 pt/10 cup dish. Heat, uncovered, on Full for 1 minute. Mix in the onions. Cook, uncovered, on Full for 5 minutes. Stir in all the remaining ingredients. Cover with clingfilm (plastic wrap) and slit it twice to allow steam to escape. Cook on Full for 15 minutes, turning the dish four times. Allow to stand for 2 minutes. Fork round lightly and serve.

Cottage Cheese and Rice Casserole

Serves 3–4

A great amalgam of tastes and textures brought back from North America some years ago.

225 g/8 oz/1 cup brown rice
50 g/2 oz/¼ cup wild rice
1.25 litre/2¼ pts/5½ cups boiling water
10 ml/2 tsp salt
4 spring onions (scallions), coarsely chopped
1 small green chilli, seeded and chopped
4 tomatoes, blanched, skinned and sliced
125 g/4 oz button mushrooms, sliced
225 g/8 oz/1 cup cottage cheese
75 g/3 oz/¾ cup Cheddar cheese, grated

Put the brown and wild rice in a 2.25 litre/4 pt/10 cup dish. Stir in the water and salt. Cover with clingfilm (plastic wrap) and slit it twice to allow steam to escape. Cook on Full for 40–45 minutes until the rice is plump and tender. Drain, if necessary, and set aside. Fill a 1.75 litre/3 pt/7½ cup casserole dish (Dutch oven) with alternate layers of rice, onions, chilli, tomatoes, mushrooms and cottage cheese. Sprinkle thickly with the grated Cheddar. Cook, uncovered, on Full for 7 minutes, turning the dish twice.

Italian Risotto

Serves 2–3

2.5–5 ml/½–1 tsp saffron powder or 5 ml/1 tsp saffron strands
50 g/2 oz/¼ cup butter
5 ml/1 tsp olive oil
1 large onion, peeled and grated
225 g/8 oz/1 cup easy-cook risotto rice
600 ml/1 pt/2½ cups boiling water or chicken stock
150 ml/¼ pt/2/3 cup dry white wine
5 ml/1 tsp salt
50 g/2 oz/½ cup grated Parmesan cheese

If using saffron strands, crumble them between your fingers into an egg cup of hot water and allow to stand for 10–15 minutes. Put half the butter and the oil in a 1.75 litre/3 pt/7½ cup dish. Heat, uncovered, on Defrost for 1 minute. Stir in the onion. Cook, uncovered, on Full for 5 minutes. Stir in the rice, water or stock and wine and either the saffron strands with the water,or the saffron powder. Cover with clingfilm (plastic wrap) and slit it twice to allow steam to escape. Cook on Full for 14 minutes, turning the dish three times. Gently fork in the remaining butter, followed by the salt and half the Parmesan cheese. Cook, uncovered, on Full for 4–8 minutes, stirring gently with a fork every 2 minutes, until the rice has absorbed all the liquid. The cooking time will depend on the rice used. Spoon into dishes and sprinkle the remaining cheese on top.

Mushroom Risotto

Serves 2–3

Break 20 g/1 oz dried mushrooms, porcini for preference, into smallish pieces, wash thoroughly under cold running water and then soak them for 10 minutes in the boiling water or chicken stock used in the Italian Risotto recipe. Proceed as for Italian Risotto.

Brazilian Rice

Serves 3–4

15 ml/1 tbsp olive or corn oil
30 ml/2 tbsp dried onion
225 g/8 oz/1 cup American long-grain or basmati rice
5–10 ml/1–2 tsp salt
600 ml/1 pt/2½ cups boiling water
2 large tomatoes, blanched, skinned and chopped

Pour the oil in a 2 litre/3½ pt/8½ cup dish. Add the dried onion. Cook, uncovered, on Full for 1¼ minutes. Stir in all the remaining ingredients. Cover with clingfilm (plastic wrap) and slit it twice to allow steam to escape. Cook on Full for 15 minutes, turning the dish four times. Allow to stand for 2 minutes. Fork round lightly and serve.

Spanish Rice

Serves 6

A North American special that has little to do with Spain other than the addition of peppers and tomatoes! Eat with poultry and egg dishes.

225 g/8 oz/1 cup easy-cook long-grain rice
600 ml/1 pt/2½ cups boiling water
10 ml/2 tsp salt
30 ml/2 tbsp corn or sunflower oil
2 onions, finely chopped
1 green (bell) pepper, seeded and coarsely chopped
400 g/14 oz/1 large can chopped tomatoes

Cook the rice in the water with half the salt as directed. Keep hot. Pour the oil into a 1.75 litre/3 pt/7½ cup bowl. Heat, uncovered, on Full for 1 minute. Stir in the onions and pepper. Cook, uncovered, on Full for 5 minutes, stirring twice. Mix in the tomatoes. Heat, uncovered, on Full for 3½ minutes. Fork in the hot rice with the remaining salt and serve straight away.

Plain Turkish Pilaf

Serves 4

225 g/8 oz/1 cup easy-cook risotto rice
Boiling water or vegetable stock
5 ml/1 tsp salt
40 g/1½ oz/3 tbsp butter

Cook the rice in the boiling water or stock with the salt added as directed. Add the butter to the dish or bowl. Allow to stand for 10 minutes. Uncover and fork round. Cover with a plate and reheat on Full for 3 minutes.

Rich Turkish Pilaf

Serves 4

225 g/8 oz/1 cup easy-cook risotto rice
Boiling water
5 ml/1 tsp salt
5 cm/2 in piece cinnamon stick
40 g/1½ oz/3 tbsp butter
15 ml/1 tbsp olive oil
2 onions, finely chopped
60 ml/4 tbsp toasted pine nuts
25 g/1 oz lambs' or chicken liver, cut into small pieces
30 ml/2 tbsp currants or raisins
2 tomatoes, blanched, skinned and chopped

Cook the rice in the water and salt, in a large dish or bowl, as directed with the cinnamon stick added. Set aside. Put the butter and oil in a 1.25 litre/2¼ pt/5½ cup bowl and heat, uncovered, on Full for 1 minute. Mix in all the remaining ingredients. Cover with a plate and cook on Full for 5 minutes, stirring twice. Stir gently into the hot rice with a fork. Cover as before and reheat on Full for 2 minutes.

Thai Rice with Lemon Grass, Lime Leaves and Coconut

Serves 4

A marvel of exquisite delicacy, appropriate for all Thai-style chicken and fish dishes.

250 g/9 oz/generous 1 cup Thai rice
400 ml/14 fl oz/1¾ cups canned coconut milk
2 fresh lime leaves
1 blade lemon grass, split lengthways, or 15 ml/1 tbsp chopped lemon balm leaves
7.5 ml/1½ tsp salt

Tip the rice into a 1.5 litre/2½ pt/6 cup dish. Pour the coconut milk into a measuring jug and make up to 600 ml/1 pt/2½ cups with cold water. Heat, uncovered, on Full for 7 minutes until it begins to bubble and boil. Stir gently into the rice with all the remaining ingredients. Cover with clingfilm (plastic wrap) and slit it twice to allow steam to escape. Cook on Full for 14 minutes. Allow to stand for 5 minutes. Uncover and remove the lemon grass, if used. Fork round gently and eat the slightly soft and sticky rice straight away.

Okra with Cabbage

Serves 6

A curiosity from the Gabon, mild or hot depending on the amount of chilli included.

30 ml/2 tbsp groundnut (peanut) oil
450 g/1 lb Savoy cabbage or spring greens (collard greens), finely shredded
200 g/7 oz okra (ladies' fingers), topped, tailed and cut into chunks
1 onion, grated
300 ml/½ pt/1¼ cups boiling water
10 ml/2 tsp salt
45 ml/3 tbsp pine nuts, lightly toasted under the grill (broiler)
2.5–20 ml/¼–4 tsp chilli powder

Pour the oil into a 2.25 litre/4 pt/10 cup casserole dish (Dutch oven). Stir in the greens and okra followed by the remaining ingredients. Mix well. Cover with clingfilm (plastic wrap) and slit it twice to allow steam to escape. Cook on Full for 7 minutes. Allow to stand for for 5 minutes. Cook on Full for a further 3 minutes. Drain if necessary and serve.

Red Cabbage with Apple

Serves 8

Magnificent with hot gammon, goose and duck, red cabbage is of Scandinavian and North European descent, a sweet-sour and now quite smart side dish, on its best behaviour in the microwave where it stays a deep rosy colour.

900 g/2 lb red cabbage
450 ml/¾ pt/2 cups boiling water
7.5 ml/1½ tsp salt
3 onions, finely chopped
3 cooking (tart) apples, peeled and grated
30 ml/2 tbsp light soft brown sugar
2.5 ml/½ tsp caraway seeds
30 ml/2 tbsp cornflour (cornstarch)
45 ml/3 tbsp malt vinegar
15 ml/1 tbsp cold water

Trim the cabbage, removing any bruised or damaged outer leaves. Cut into quarters and remove the hard central stalk, then shred as finely as possible. Put into a 2.25 litre/4 pt/10 cup dish. Add half the boiling water and 5 ml/1 tsp of the salt. Cover with a plate and cook on Full for 10 minutes, turning the dish four times. Stir well, then mix in the remaining boiling water and remaining salt, the onions, apples, sugar and caraway seeds. Cover with clingfilm (plastic wrap) and slit it twice to allow steam to escape. Cook on Full for 20 minutes, turning the dish four times. Remove from the microwave. Mix the cornflour smoothly with the vinegar and cold water. Add to the hot cabbage and mix well. Cook, uncovered, on Full for 10 minutes, stirring three times. Leave until cold before chilling overnight. To serve, re-cover with fresh clingfilm and slit it twice to allow steam to escape, then heat on Full for 5–6 minutes before serving. Alternatively, transfer portions to side plates and cover each with kitchen paper, then reheat individually on Full for 1 minute each.

Red Cabbage with Wine

Serves 8

Prepare as for Red Cabbage with Apples, but substitute 250 ml/8 fl oz/1 cup red wine for half the boiling water.

Norwegian Sour Cabbage

Serves 8

900 g/2 lb white cabbage
90 ml/6 tbsp water
60 ml/4 tbsp malt vinegar
60 ml/4 tbsp granulated sugar
10 ml/2 tsp caraway seeds
7.5–10 ml/1½–2 tsp salt

Trim the cabbage, removing any bruised or damaged outer leaves. Cut into quarters and remove the hard central stalk, then shred as finely as possible. Put into a 2.25 litre/4 pt/10 cup dish with all the remaining ingredients. Mix thoroughly with two spoons. Cover with clingfilm (plastic wrap) and slit it twice to allow steam to escape. Cook on Defrost for 45 minutes, turning the dish four times. Leave at kitchen temperature overnight for the flavours to mature. To serve, put individual servings on to side plates and cover each with kitchen paper. Reheat individually on Full, allowing about 1 minute each. Securely cover and then refrigerate any leftovers.

Greek-style Stewed Okra with Tomatoes

Serves 6–8

Very marginally Eastern in character, this slightly off-beat vegetable dish has become a viable proposition now that okra (ladies' fingers) is more widely available. This recipe is excellent with lamb or as a dish in its own right, served with rice.

900 g/2 lb okra, topped and tailed
Salt and freshly ground black pepper
90 ml/6 tbsp malt vinegar
45 ml/3 tbsp olive oil
2 onions, peeled and finely chopped
6 tomatoes, blanched, skinned and coarsely chopped
15 ml/1 tbsp light soft brown sugar

Spread out the okra on a large flat plate. To reduce the chances of the okra splitting and taking on a slimy feel, sprinkle with salt and the vinegar. Allow to stand for for 30 minutes. Wash and wipe dry on kitchen paper. Pour the oil into a 2.5 litre/4½ pt/11 cup dish and add the onions. Cook, uncovered, on Full for 7 minutes, stirring three times. Stir in all the remaining ingredients including the okra and season to taste. Cover with a plate and cook on Full for 9–10 minutes, stirring three or four times, until the okra is tender. Allow to stand for 3 minutes before serving.

Greens with Tomatoes, Onions and Peanut Butter

Serves 4–6

Try this Malawi speciality with sliced white bread as a vegetarian main course or serve as a side dish with chicken.

450 g/1 lb spring greens (collard greens), finely shredded
150 ml/¼ pt/2/3 cup boiling water
5–7.5 ml/1–1½ tsp salt
4 tomatoes, blanched, skinned and sliced
1 large onion, finely chopped
60 ml/4 tbsp crunchy peanut butter

Place the greens in a 2.25 litre/4 pt/10 cup dish. Mix in the water and salt. Cover with clingfilm (plastic wrap) and slit it twice to allow steam to escape. Cook on Full for 20 minutes. Uncover and stir in the tomatoes, onion and peanut butter. Cover as before and cook on Full for 5 minutes.

Sweet-sour Creamed Beetroot

Serves 4

This attractive way of presenting beetroot dates back to 1890, but it's currently back in fashion.

450 g/1 lb cooked beetroot (red beets), coarsely grated
150 ml/¼ pt/2/3 cup double (heavy) cream
Salt
15 ml/1 tbsp vinegar
30 ml/2 tbsp demerara sugar

Put the beetroot in a 900 ml/1½ pt/3¾ cup dish with the cream and salt to taste. Cover with a plate and heat through on Full for 3 minutes, stirring once. Stir in the vinegar and sugar and serve straight away.

Beetroot in Orange

Serves 4–6

A lively and original accompaniment to Christmas meats and poultry.

450 g/1 lb cooked beetroot (red beets), peeled and sliced
75 ml/5 tbsp freshly squeezed orange juice
15 ml/1 tbsp malt vinegar
2.5 ml/½ tsp salt
1 garlic clove, peeled and crushed

Place the beetroot in a shallow 18 cm/7 in diameter dish. Beat together the remaining ingredients and pour over the beetroot. Cover with clingfilm (plastic wrap) and slit it twice to allow steam to escape. Cook on Full for 6 minutes, turning the dish three times. Allow to stand for 1 minute.

Scalloped Celeriac

Serves 6

A handsome and gourmet-style winter side dish that teams happily with fish and poultry.

4 lean rashers (slices) bacon, chopped
900 g/2 lb celeriac (celery root)
300 ml/½ pt/1¼ cups cold water
15 ml/1 tbsp lemon juice
7.5 ml/1½ tsp salt
300 ml/½ pt/1¼ cups single (light) cream
1 small bag potato crisps (chips), crushed in the bag

Put the bacon on a plate and cover with kitchen paper. Cook on Full for 3 minutes. Peel the celeriac thickly, wash well and cut each head into eight pieces. Place in a 2.25 litre/4 pt/10 cup dish with the water, lemon juice and salt. Cover with clingfilm (plastic wrap) and slit it twice to allow steam to escape. Cook on Full for 20 minutes, turning the dish four times. Drain. Slice the celeriac and return to the dish. Stir in the bacon and cream and sprinkle with the crisps. Cook, uncovered, on Full for 4 minutes, turning the dish twice. Allow to stand for 5 minutes before serving.

Celeriac with Orange Hollandaise Sauce

Serves 6

Celeriac with a gloriously golden, gleaming topping of citrus Hollandaise sauce to try with duck and game.

900 g/2 lb celeriac (celery root)
300 ml/½ pt/1¼ cups cold water
15 ml/1 tbsp lemon juice
7.5 ml/1½ tsp salt
Maltese Sauce
1 very sweet orange, peeled and segmented

Peel the celeriac thickly, wash well and cut each head into eight pieces. Place in a 2.25 litre/4 pt/10 cup dish with the water, lemon juice and salt. Cover with clingfilm (plastic wrap) and slit it twice to allow steam to escape. Cook on Full for 20 minutes, turning the dish four times. Drain. Slice the celeriac and return to the dish. Keep hot. Make the Maltese Sauce and spoon over the celeriac. Garnish with the orange segments.

Slimmers' Vegetable Pot

Serves 2

Prepare as for Slimmer's Fish Pot but omit the fish. Add the diced flesh of 2 avocados to the cooked vegetables with the spices and herbs. Cover and reheat on Full for 1½ minutes.

Slimmers' Vegetable Pot with Eggs

Serves 2

Prepare as for Slimmer's Vegetable Pot, but sprinkle each portion with 1 chopped hard-boiled (hard-cooked) egg.

Ratatouille

Serves 6–8

An explosion of Mediterranean flavours and colours is part and parcel of this glorious vegetable pot-pourri. Hot, cold or warm – it seems to go with everything.

60 ml/4 tbsp olive oil
3 onions, peeled and coarsely chopped
1–3 garlic cloves, crushed
225 g/8 oz courgettes (zucchini), thinly sliced
350 g/12 oz/3 cups cubed aubergine (eggplant)
1 large red or green (bell) pepper, seeded and chopped
3 ripe tomatoes, skinned, blanched and chopped
30 ml/2 tbsp tomato purée (paste)
20 ml/4 tsp light soft brown sugar
10 ml/2 tsp salt
45–60 ml/3–4 tbsp chopped parsley

Pour the oil into a 2.5 litre/4½ pt/11 cup dish. Heat, uncovered, on Full for 1 minute. Mix in the onions and garlic. Cook, uncovered, on Full for 4 minutes. Stir in all the remaining ingredients except half the parsley. Cover with a plate and cook on Full for 20 minutes, stirring three or four times. Uncover and cook on Full for 8–10 minutes, stirring four times, until most of the liquid has evaporated. Mix in the remaining parsley. Serve straight away or cool, cover and chill if to be eaten later.

Caramelised Parsnips

Serves 4

Ideal with all poultry and beef roasts, choose baby parsnips no bigger than large carrots for this.

450 g/1 lb small parsnips, thinly sliced
45 ml/3 tbsp water
25 g/1 oz/2 tbsp butter
7.5 ml/1½ tbsp dark soft brown sugar
Salt

Put the parsnips in a 1.25 litre/2¼ pt/5½ cup dish with the water. Cover with clingfilm (plastic wrap) and slit it twice to allow steam to escape. Cook on Full for 8–10 minutes, turning the dish and gently shaking the contents twice, until tender. Drain off the water. Add the butter and sugar and toss the parsnips to coat them thoroughly. Heat, uncovered, on Full for 1–1½ minutes until glazed. Sprinkle with salt and eat straight away.

Parsnips with Egg and Butter Crumb Sauce

Serves 4

450 g/1 lb parsnips, diced
45 ml/3 tbsp water
75 g/3 oz/1/3 cup unsalted (sweet) butter
4 spring onions (scallions), finely chopped
45 ml/3 tbsp light-coloured toasted breadcrumbs
1 hard-boiled (hard-cooked) egg, grated
30 ml/2 tbsp finely chopped parsley
Juice of ½ small lemon

Place the parsnips in a 1.5 litre/2½ pt/6 cup dish with the water. Cover with clingfilm (plastic wrap) and slit it twice to allow steam to escape. Cook on Full for 8–10 minutes. Allow to stand while preparing the sauce. Put the butter in a measuring jug and melt, uncovered, on Defrost for 2–2½ minutes. Stir in the onions and cook, uncovered, on Defrost for 3 minutes, stirring twice. Mix in all the remaining ingredients and heat on Defrost for 30 seconds. Drain the parsnips and transfer to a warmed serving dish. Coat with the crumb sauce and serve straight away.

Chocolate Fondue

Serves 3–4

200 g/7 oz plain (semi-sweet) chocolate
150 ml/¼ pt/2/3 cup double (heavy) cream
15 ml/1 tbsp whisky, rum, brandy or orange-flavoured liqueur or 5 ml/1 tsp vanilla essence (extract)
Small biscuits, marshmallows and/or pieces of fresh fruit, to serve

Break up the chocolate and place in a basin. Melt, uncovered, on Defrost for 4–5 minutes until soft. Stir in the cream and heat, uncovered, on Defrost for about 1½ minutes. Stir in the alcohol or vanilla essence. Serve warm with biscuits, marshmallows and/or fresh fruit pieces for dipping.

Orange Chocolate Fondue

Serves 3–4

Prepare as for Chocolate Fondue, but use only Grand Marnier, Mandarine Napolean liqueur or Cointreau. Flavour with 5 ml/1 tsp finely grated orange peel.

Mocha Fondue

Serves 3–4

Prepare as for Chocolate Fondue, but add 15 ml/1 tbsp instant coffee powder with the cream and use only Tia Maria, Kahlua or coffee essence (extract) to flavour.

White Chocolate Fondue

Serves 3–4

Prepare as for Chocolate Fondue, but substitute white chocolate for the plain (semi-sweet) and add 30 ml/2 tbsp of the measured cream to the chocolate before melting. Flavour with vanilla essence (extract) or an orange liqueur instead of the suggested spirits.

Toblerone Fondue

Serves 3–4

Prepare as for Chocolate Fondue, but substitute white, milk or dark Toblerone chocolate for the plain (semi-sweet) chocolate.

Royal Chocolate Mousse

Makes 10–12

15 ml/1 tbsp powdered gelatine
150 ml/¼ pt/2/3 cup cold water
500 g/1 lb 2 oz plain (semi-sweet) chocolate (70% cocoa)
30 ml/2 tbsp butter
75 ml/3 fl oz/5½ tbsp strong hot coffee
4 eggs, at kitchen temperature, separated
A pinch of salt
Coffee or cocoa (unsweetened chocolate) powder, to serve

Soak the gelatine in a glass jug in cold water 5 minutes. Melt, uncovered, on Full for 1½–2 minutes until the liquid looks clear. Stir round, then set aside. Break up the chocolate and place in a fairly large bowl with the butter and coffee. Melt, uncovered, on Defrost for 6–7 minutes. Stir in the egg yolks and melted gelatine. Chill until just beginning to thicken and set slightly round the edges. Whisk together the egg whites and salt until they form stiff peaks. Beat one-third into the chocolate mixture, then gently and smoothly fold in the remainder. Divide between 10–12 ramekin dishes (custard cups). Chill for several hours until firm. Dust with coffee or cocoa powder before serving.

Dutch-style Pears with Chocolate Advocaat Mousse

Serves 6

10 ml/2 tsp powdered gelatine
30 ml/2 tbsp cold water
100 g/3½ oz plain (semi-sweet) chocolate
2 eggs, at kitchen temperature, separated
150 ml/¼ pt/2/3 cup advocaat (egg liqueur)
425 g/15 oz/1 large can pear halves in juice or syrup, drained
30 ml/2 tbsp chopped pistachio nuts

Soak the gelatine in a glass jug in cold water for 5 minutes. Melt, uncovered, on Full for 1–1½ minutes until the liquid looks clear. Stir round and set aside. Break up the chocolate and place in a separate bowl. Melt, uncovered, on Defrost for 3–3½ minutes. Stir well. Mix in the dissolved gelatine, egg yolks and advocaat. Beat until smooth and evenly combined. Cover and chill until just beginning to thicken and set. Beat the egg whites to stiff peaks. Whisk one-third into the chocolate mixture, then fold in the remainder with a metal spoon. Divide the pears between six sundae glasses and top evenly with the chocolate mixture. Chill until set. Sprinkle with the nuts before serving.

Traditional Chocolate Mousse

Serves 4

100 g/3½ oz plain (semi-sweet) chocolate
15 ml/1 tbsp unsalted (sweet) butter
4 eggs at kitchen temperature, separated
A pinch of salt
Sponge finger biscuits (cookies), to serve

Break up chocolate, then put in a 1.25 litre/2¼ pt/5½ cup basin with the butter. Heat, uncovered, on Defrost for 3½–4 minutes, stirring once or twice, until both have melted. Mix in the egg yolks. In a separate bowl, beat the egg whites and salt to stiff peaks. Beat one-third into the chocolate mixture, then smoothly stir in the remainder with a large metal spoon. Spoon into four stemmed wine glasses. Cover with kitchen paper and chill thoroughly. Eat with sponge fingers.

Chocolate Orange Mousse

Serves 4

Prepare as for Traditional Chocolate Mousse, but add 10 ml/2 tsp finely grated orange peel with the egg yolks.

Mocha Mousse

Serves 4

Prepare as for Traditional Chocolate Mousse, but add 10 ml/2 tsp instant coffee granules with the egg yolks.

Chocolate Peppermint Cream Mousse

Serves 4

Prepare as for Traditional Chocolate Mousse, but add a few drops of peppermint essence (extract) with the egg yolks. Just before serving, decorate the top of each with whipped cream.

Berlin Air

Serves 6–8

Germany's answer to Italy's zabaglione and Britain's syllabub.

4 large eggs, separated
A pinch of salt
150 g/5 oz/2/3 cup caster (superfine) sugar
5 ml/1 tsp vanilla essence (extract)
10 ml/2 tsp cornflour (cornstarch)
150 ml/¼ pt/2/3 cup sweet white wine
150 ml/¼ pt/2/3 cup double (heavy) cream
30 ml/2 tbsp brandy
Wafer biscuits (cookies) and mixed berry fruits (optional), to serve

Whisk the egg whites with the salt until stiff. Whisk together the yolks, sugar and vanilla in a large bowl until the mixture is pale and thick. Gently whisk in the whites. Mix the cornflour smoothly with a little of the wine, then stir in the remainder. Fold into the egg mixture. Cook, uncovered, on Full for 3½ minutes, whisking every 30 seconds, until the mixture is foaming and resembles thickish custard. Cover and leave until completely cold. In large bowl, whisk the cream with the brandy until thick. Gradually whisk in the egg mixture. Spoon into six to eight individual ramekin dishes (custard cups) and chill thoroughly. Serve with crisp wafer biscuits and accompany, in season, with fresh berry fruits.

Crème Caramel

Serves 4

Prepare one quantity of Baked Egg Custard. Pour bought caramel sauce into four buttered ramekin dishes (custard cups) and top with the egg custard. Cook, uncovered, on Defrost for 8–9 minutes until the custard is set. Allow to cool, then chill thoroughly. Turn out on to individual plates and serve with cream.

Spicy Peaches and Oranges in Red Wine

Serves 6–8

8 large ripe peaches, blanched and skinned
Lemon juice
300 ml/½ pt/1¼ cups dry red wine
175 g/6 oz/¾ cup caster (superfine) sugar
5 cm/2 in piece cinnamon stick
4 whole cloves
2 cardamom pods
2 oranges, unpeeled and thinly sliced

Halve the peaches and twist to separate. Remove the stones (pits). Brush the flesh all over with lemon juice. Put the remaining ingredients except the oranges in a deep 20 cm/8 in diameter dish. Cover with an inverted plate and heat on Full for 4 minutes. Stir to mix. Add the peaches, cut sides down, and arrange the orange slices randomly between. Cover with clingfilm (plastic wrap) and slit it twice to allow steam to escape. Cook on Full for 10 minutes, turning the dish twice. Cool and chill before serving.

Spicy Pears and Oranges in Red Wine

Serves 6–8

Prepare as for Spicy Peaches and Oranges in Red Wine, but substitute 8 small dessert pears, peeled, halved and cored, for the peaches.

Store-cupboard Raspberry Mousse

Serves 6

15 ml/1 tbsp powdered gelatine
30 ml/2 tbsp cold water
425 g/15 oz/1 large can raspberries in syrup, drained and syrup reserved
3 eggs, separated
45 ml/3 tbsp caster (superfine) sugar
A pinch of salt
150 ml/¼ pt/2/3 cup whipping cream
15 ml/1 tbsp toasted and chopped hazelnuts, to decorate

Put the gelatine in a jug with the cold water. Stir round and leave for 5 minutes to soften. Melt, uncovered, on Full for 2 minutes until the liquid is clear. Add the raspberry syrup to the gelatine. Gently beat in the egg yolks and sugar. Cover and chill until just beginning to thicken and set. Beat the egg whites and salt until stiff. Whip the cream until thick. Beat one-third of the egg whites into the gelatine mixture, then mix in two-thirds of the raspberries and three-quarters of the cream. Fold in the remaining whites with a metal spoon. When smooth and well-combined, transfer to six dessert dishes. Cover and chill until set. Before serving, stir the remaining cream into the remaining raspberries and use to decorate the top of the mousses.

Egg Custard, Apricot and Sherry Trifle

Serves 8

600 ml/1 pt/2½ cups full-cream milk or half single (light) cream and half milk
15 ml/1 tbsp cornflour (cornstarch)
15 ml/1 tbsp cold water
4 large eggs
75 ml/5 tbsp caster (superfine) sugar
5 ml/1 tsp vanilla essence (extract)
2 jam (conserve)-filled Swiss (jelly) rolls, thinly sliced
425 g/15 oz/1 large can apricot halves, drained
30 ml/2 tbsp sweet sherry
60 ml/4 tbsp apricot syrup
150 ml/¼ pt/2/3 cup double (heavy) cream
Hundreds and thousands, to decorate

Pour the milk into a jug. Warm, uncovered, on Full for 2 minutes. Put the cornflour and water in a 1.25 litre/2¼ pt/5½ cup bowl and stir until smooth. Beat in the eggs one at a time. Add 45 ml/3 tbsp of the caster sugar and mix in the warm milk. Cook, uncovered, on Full for 5–6 minutes, whisking every minute, until the custard is of a thin coating consistency (it thickens on cooling). Mix in the vanilla. Cover and set aside. Stand eight slices of Swiss roll against the side of a deep 20 cm/8 in diameter glass serving dish. Reserve 8 apricot halves for decoration and coarsely chop the remainder. Use to cover the base of the dish with the remaining Swiss roll. Moisten with the sherry and apricot syrup. Coat with half the warm custard and let it soak well in. Pour the remaining custard over the top. Cover and chill for 4–5 hours. Before serving, beat together the cream and remaining caster sugar until thick. Use to decorate the top of the trifle, then arrange the reserved apricot halves on top. Dust with hundreds and thousands.

Short-cut Sherry Trifle

Serves 6–8

1 jam (conserve)-filled Swiss (jelly) roll, thinly sliced
45 ml/3 tbsp sweet sherry
425 g/15 oz/1 large can peach slices or fruit cocktail, drained and syrup reserved
45 ml/3 tbsp custard powder
30 ml/2 tbsp caster (superfine) sugar
600 ml/1 pt/2½ cups cold milk
150 ml/¼ pt/2/3 cup whipped cream
Hundreds and thousands and red glacé (candied) cherries

Arrange the Swiss roll slices over the base and half-way up the side of a shallow glass bowl. Moisten with the sherry and few spoonfuls of the reserved syrup. Cover with the drained fruit. Put the custard powder and sugar in a fairly deep dish and mix smoothly with a little of the cold milk. Blend in the remainder. Cook, uncovered, on Full for 8 minutes, whisking briskly every minute to keep the custard smooth. Allow to cool slightly, then pour over the trifle. Cover when cold and chill thoroughly. Before serving, decorate with the whipped cream, hundreds and thousands and glacé cherries.

Note: use up any left-over syrup in fresh fruit salad.

Chocolate Cream Trifle

Serves 8

Prepare as for Egg Custard, Apricot and Sherry Trifle, but use 2 cream-filled chocolate Swiss (jelly) rolls instead of jam-filled. Substitute coffee liqueur for the sherry and canned pear halves for the apricots. Sprinkle with grated chocolate or a crushed flake bar instead of the hundreds and thousands.

Trifle with Sponge Cakes

Serves 6–8

Make any of the three trifles above, but substitute bought sponge cakes (8 in a packet) for the Swiss (jelly) roll. Split and fill with jam (conserve), curd or chocolate spread.

Fluffy Lemon Clouds

Serves 4–5

300 ml/½ pt/1¼ cups cold milk
25 ml/1½ tbsp custard powder
15 ml/1 tbsp caster (superfine) sugar
2 large eggs, separated
1 packet lemon jelly (jello)
A pinch of salt
Seasonal fruits, to decorate

Blend some of the cold milk smoothly with the custard powder in a large bowl. Mix in the remainder. Cook, uncovered, on Full for 3–3½ minutes, whisking every minute to prevent lumps forming, until the mixture comes to the boil and thickens. Beat in the sugar and egg yolks. Cover with a piece of clingfilm (plastic wrap), placing it directly on the surface of the custard to stop a skin forming. Allow to cool. Break up the jelly into cubes. Put in a measuring jug with 60 ml/4 tbsp water. Cover with a saucer and melt on Defrost for 2–2½ minutes, stirring twice. Make up to 300 ml/½ pt/1¼ cups with cold water. Lift the clingfilm off the custard and beat in the melted jelly. Cover and chill until the mixture is beginning to thicken and set. Whisk the egg whites and salt until stiff. Beat one-third into the jelly mixture, then smoothly fold in the remainder with a large metal spoon or balloon whisk. Transfer to four or five dessert glasses or dishes. Cover and chill until firm and set. Decorate with fresh seasonal fruits.

Fluffy Lime Clouds

Serves 4–5

Prepare as for Fluffy Lemon Clouds, but substitute lime jelly (jello) for the lemon.

Apple Snow

Serves 4

30 ml/2 tbsp vanilla-flavoured blancmange powder
450 ml/¾ pt/2 cups cold milk
45 ml/3 tbsp caster (superfine) sugar
125 g/4 oz/½ cup smooth apple purée (apple sauce)
2 large eggs, separated
A squeeze of lemon juice
Grated lemon peel

Tip the blancmange powder into a 1.75 litre/3 pt/7½ cup bowl. Mix smoothly with 60 ml/4 tbsp of the measured milk. Pour the remaining milk into a basin. Heat, uncovered, on Full for 4 minutes. Blend into the blancmange mixture. Add the sugar and stir thoroughly. Cook, uncovered, on Full for about 2½ minutes, beating every minute, until smooth and thickened. Whisk in the apple purée and egg yolks. Cover and allow to cool to lukewarm. Beat together the egg whites and lemon juice to stiff peaks. Whisk one-third into the blancmange mixture, then gently fold in the remainder with a large metal spoon.

Spoon into four dishes or glasses. Cover and chill for several hours. Sprinkle each lightly with lemon peel before serving.

Apricot Snow

Serves 4

Prepare as for Apple Snow, but substitute apricot purée (sauce) for the apple purée.

Lemon Meringue Spiced Pears

Serves 6

Altogether a surprise package.

75 g/3 oz/1/3 cup light soft brown sugar
300 ml/½ pt/1¼ cups water
60 ml/4 tbsp dry white wine
5 cm/2 inch piece cinnamon stick
4 whole cloves
6 firm dessert pears
1 packet lemon meringue filling mix
150 ml/¼ pt/2/3 cup milk, at kitchen temperature
Finely grated peel of 1 small lemon
Basil leaves, to decorate

Put the sugar, water, wine, cinnamon stick and cloves in a 1.75 litre/3 pt/7½ cup dish. Heat, uncovered, on Full for 3 minutes. Set aside. Peel the pears, leaving the stalks in place. Arrange upright in the dish and baste with the spicy syrup mixture. Slide the dish into a roasting bag and tie up with string. Cook on Full for 7 minutes. Remove from the microwave and take the dish from the bag. Carefully strain the syrup into a measuring jug. Stir in the lemon filling mix. Cover with saucer and cook on Full for 2–3 minutes, whisking every 30 seconds, until the mixture comes to the boil. Allow to cool for 5 minutes. Whisk in the milk and lemon peel. Cover and chill both the pears and the lemon sauce for several hours. Before serving, coat the pears with about half the sauce and decorate with basil leaves. Pour the remainder into a jug and pass separately.

Finnish Cranberry Whip

Serves 6

225 g/8 oz cranberries, thawed if frozen
150 ml/¼ pt/2/3 cup water
175 g/6 oz/¾ cup caster (superfine) sugar
5 ml/1 tsp finely grated lemon peel
150 ml/¼ pt/2/3 cup whipping cream
150 ml/¼ pt/2/3 cup double (heavy) cream
2 large egg whites

Put the cranberries, water, sugar and lemon peel in a 1.25 litre/2¼ pt/5½ cup dish. Cover with a plate and cook on Full for 8½ minutes, stirring twice and crushing the fruit against the side of the dish. Allow to cool completely. Whip the creams together until thick. Beat the egg whites to stiff peaks. Fold the cream and egg whites alternately into the cranberries. Transfer to six individual dishes. Chill lightly before serving.

Cranberry and Orange Whip

Serves 6

Prepare as for Finnish Cranberry Whip, but add 10 ml/2 tsp grated orange peel with the lemon peel.

Kissel

Serves 4

Russia's answer to blancmange, made from fruits growing wild in the countryside around country dachas or wooden holiday homes.

450 g/1 lb mixed soft berry fruits
60 ml/4 tbsp red wine, apple juice or water
75 g/3 oz/1/3 cup caster (superfine) sugar
5 ml/1 tsp vanilla essence (extract)
Peel of 1 lemon, cut into strips
15 ml/1 tbsp cornflour (cornstarch) or potato flour
30 ml/2 tbsp cold water
Single (light) cream or Home-made Yoghurt, to serve

Purée the fruit in a blender or food processor. Sieve to remove the seeds. Pour the wine, juice or water into a mixing bowl. Add the sugar, vanilla and lemon strips. Cover with a plate and cook on Full for 3½ minutes, stirring twice to ensure the sugar has dissolved. Add the berry purée. Cover as before and cook on Full for 2 minutes. Strain into a clean bowl. Blend the cornflour or potato flour smoothly with the water. Add to the fruit mixture. Cook, uncovered, on Full for 2–3 minutes, stirring three times, until thickened. Allow to cool slightly. Transfer to four dessert dishes, then cover and chill for several hours. Float cream or yoghurt over the top of each before serving.

Home-made Yoghurt

Makes about 900 ml/1½ pt/3¾ cups

900 ml/1½ pts/3¾ cups full-cream milk
60 ml/4 tbsp skimmed milk powder (non-fat dry milk)
150 ml/¼ pt/2/3 cup plain yoghurt

Pour the milk into a bowl. Heat, uncovered, on Defrost for about 4–5 minutes until lukewarm but not hot. Whisk in the skimmed milk and yoghurt. Cover. Leave to stand in a warm place for 12 hours until set – a linen cupboard is ideal. Store in the refrigerator when cold.

Apricot Pots

Serves 8

350 g/12 oz/2 cups dried apricot halves
600 ml/1 pt/2½ cups boiling water
30 ml/2 tbsp orange flower water
60 ml/4 tbsp icing (confectioners') sugar, sifted
225 g/8 oz/1 cup thick Greek-style plain yoghurt
Raspberry Coulis

Thoroughly wash the apricots, then soak in boiling water, covered with a plate, for at least 6 hours. Drain and transfer to a bowl. Add the measured boiling water. Cover with clingfilm (plastic wrap) and slit it twice to allow steam to escape. Cook on Defrost for 25–30 minutes, turning the bowl three times. Remove from the microwave and allow to cool to lukewarm. Tip into a food processor with the orange flower water and sugar and run the machine until the mixture forms a fairly smooth purée. Combine with the yoghurt and spoon evenly into eight ramekin dishes (custard cups). Cover and chill. Before serving, cover each with the coulis.

Prune Pots

Serves 8

350 g/12 oz dried stoned (pitted) prunes
600 ml/1 pt/2½ cups boiling water
30 ml/2 tbsp orange flower water
60 ml/4 tbsp icing (confectioners') sugar, sifted
30–45 ml/2–3 tbsp Armagnac
225 g/8 oz/1 cup thick Greek-style plain yoghurt
Chopped pecan nuts and demerara sugar, to serve

Thoroughly wash the prunes, then soak in boiling water, covered with plate, for at least 6 hours. Drain and transfer to a bowl. Add the measured boiling water. Cover with clingfilm (plastic wrap) and slit it twice to allow steam to escape. Cook on Defrost for 25–30 minutes, turning the bowl three times. Remove from the microwave and allow to cool to lukewarm. Tip the drained prunes, orange flower water, sugar and Armagnac into a food processor and run the machine until the mixture forms a fairly smooth purée. Combine with the yoghurt and spoon evenly into eight ramekin dishes (custard cups). Cover and chill. Before serving, sprinkle each with pecan nuts and demerara sugar.

Cherries Jubilee

Serves 6

One of North America's prize specimens and a show-off designed to impress.

400 g/14 oz/1 large can black cherry fruit filling
30 ml/2 tbsp cold water
30 ml/2 tbsp Kirsch or brandy
Vanilla ice cream

Put the fruit filling in a bowl and stir in the water. Heat, uncovered, on Defrost for 3 minutes. Stir round. Spread evenly into a shallow serving dish. In a separate dish, warm the spirit, uncovered, on Defrost for 45 seconds. Pour over the cherries and carefully ignite. Serve immediately over scoops of ice cream.

Fruits of the Forest Jubilee

Serves 6

Prepare as for Cherries Jubilee, but substitute apple and blackberry fruit filling for black cherry and strawberry ice cream for vanilla.

Dutch Chocolate Sundaes

Serves 4

90 ml/6 tbsp advocaat
75 ml/5 tbsp single (light) cream
2 small bananas, thinly sliced
Vanilla or chocolate ice cream
1 chocolate flake bar, crushed

Pour the advocaat into a dish and stir in the cream. Add the bananas. Heat, uncovered, on Defrost for 3 minutes. Mix gently. Spoon over scoops of ice cream in sundae dishes or dessert glasses and sprinkle with the chocolate flake. Eat straight away.

Cream Liqueur Sundaes

Serves 4

Prepare as for Dutch Chocolate Sundaes, but substitute any cream liqueur, quantity to taste, for the advocaat.

Grape and Raspberry Jelly

Serves 4

1 packet raspberry jelly (jello)
225 g/8 oz mixed black and green seedless grapes, rinsed and drained
Wafer biscuits (cookies), to serve

Snip the jelly into cubes with kitchen scissors and put in a measuring cup with 60 ml/4 tbsp cold water. Melt, uncovered, on Defrost for 2–2½ minutes. Make up to 450 ml/¾ pt/2 cups with cold water. Cover and chill until just beginning to thicken and set – it must not be at all runny. Fold the grapes into the thickened jelly with a spoon. Divide equally between four dessert dishes or stemmed glasses. Cover loosely with kitchen paper and chill until set. Serve with wafer biscuits.

Mandarin and Lemon Jelly

Serves 4

Prepare as for Grape and Raspberry Jelly, but substitute lemon jelly (jello) for the raspberry and peeled fresh mandarin, clementine or satsuma segments, halved, for the grapes.

Black Cherry Rice Cream

Serves 4

1 packet black cherry jelly (jello)
400 g/14 oz/1 large can rice pudding
75 ml/5 tbsp single (light) cream
30 ml/2 tbsp black cherry jam (conserve)

Snip the jelly into cubes with kitchen scissors and put in a measuring cup. Melt, uncovered, on Defrost for 2–2½ minutes. Fold in the rice pudding and cream, whisking gently without beating. Make up to 600 ml/1 pt/2½ cups with cold water. Cover lightly and chill until just beginning to thicken and set, stirring frequently. Divide equally between four sundae glasses and allow to set completely. Top each with 7.5 ml/1½ tsp jam before serving.

Banana Splits

Serves 4

The return of something special after a long time away.

Peel 4 large bananas, then halve each lengthways. Arrange on four plates. Put 2 scoops of vanilla ice cream in between each to make a 'sandwich', then top with any of the hot chocolate sauce recipes. Pipe or spoon on softly whipped cream and serve straight away.

Spicy Prune Froth

Serves 4

450 ml/¾ pt/2 cups prune juice
15 ml/1 tbsp powdered gelatine
8 cm/3 in piece cinnamon stick
2 star anise
30 ml/2 tbsp fine-shred orange marmalade
2 large egg whites
A pinch of salt
30 ml/2 tbsp whipped cream
Ground cinnamon

Pour 45 ml/3 tbsp of the prune juice into a small bowl. Add the gelatine and stir round. Stand for 5 minutes to soften. Melt, uncovered, on Defrost for 2–2½ minutes. Set aside. Pour the remaining prune juice into a large jug and add the cinnamon stick, star anise and marmalade. Heat, uncovered, on Full for 6 minutes or until the liquid just begins to bubble. Gently beat in the dissolved gelatine. Strain into a clean bowl. Cover with a plate and allow to cool, then chill until just beginning to thicken and set. Whisk the egg whites and salt until stiff. Beat one-third into the part-set prune jelly, then fold in the remaining whites thoroughly with large metal spoon or spatula. Spoon into four glass dishes, cover loosely and allow to set for several hours in the refrigerator. Before serving, decorate each with cream and dust with cinnamon.

Chilled Oranges with Hot Chocolate Peppermint Sauce

Serves 4

4 large oranges, peeled and very thinly sliced
Hot Chocolate Peppermint Sauce
Mint sprigs

Peel and very thinly slice the oranges, ensuring any pips (pits) are removed. Arrange on four side plates, then cover and chill until almost icy. Immediately before serving, drizzle the sauce over each, then garnish with mint sprigs.

Summer Fruit Mould

Serves 4

A sort of summer pudding in an instant. It is markedly sweet-sour and benefits from a drizzle of custard or sweetened cream.

500 g/1 lb 2 oz frozen mixed summer fruits
1 packet raspberry jelly (jello)

Tip the fruit into a bowl. Cover with a plate and thaw on Defrost for 7–8 minutes. Remove from the microwave. Snip the jelly into cubes and put in a bowl or jug. Melt, uncovered, on Defrost for 2½ minutes. Stir into the fruits. Chill until just beginning to thicken and set, stirring frequently so that the fruit stays suspended in the jelly. Transfer to a wetted mould or basin and cover. Chill until firm and completely set. Invert on to a plate and serve.

Watermelon and Apricot Chill with Frosted Grapes

Serves 4

150 ml/¼ pt/2/3 cup sweet white wine
150 ml/¼ pt/2/3 cup white grape juice
Peel of 1 lime, cut into narrow strips
175 g/6 oz/1 cup dried apricots, well washed and cut into strips
5 ml/1 tsp vanilla essence (extract)
2.5 ml/½ tsp almond essence (extract)
1 large wedge red watermelon
4 clusters black seedless grapes
1 small egg white, lightly beaten
Caster (superfine) sugar

Pour the wine and grape juice into a 1.25 litre/2¼ pt/5½ cup bowl. Add half the lime peel. Heat, uncovered, on Full for 4 minutes. Add the apricot strips. Cook, uncovered, on Full for 2 minutes. Stir in the vanilla and almond essence (extract). Cover and allow to cool. Thoroughly chill when cold. Slice the watermelon flesh away from its skin and remove all the black seeds. Cut the flesh into small cubes. Set aside. Wash and dry the grapes but leave attached to their stalks. Dip them in egg white to cover, then coat thickly with caster sugar. Leave to dry and set for at least an hour. Add the melon to the apricot mixture and transfer to four glass dessert dishes. Top each with a bunch of frosted grapes and the remaining lime peel, cut into narrow strips.

Rhubarb and Mandarin Cups

Serves 6

450 g/1 lb rhubarb, trimmed and chopped
300 gl/11 oz/1 large can mandarin oranges in syrup
60 ml/4 tbsp granulated sugar
5 ml/1 tsp finely grated orange peel
Raspberry or strawberry sorbet

Put the rhubarb in a 1.25 litre/2¼ pt/5½ cup dish with 30 ml/2 tbsp syrup from the mandarins and all the sugar. Cover with a plate and cook on Full for 7–9 minutes until the rhubarb is tender. Uncover and stir in the drained mandarins and orange peel. Cover and cool, then chill for several hours. Spoon into six glasses over scoops of sorbet and eat straight away.

Rhubarb and Mandarin Cups with Ginger Cream

Serves 6

450 g/1 lb rhubarb, trimmed and chopped
300 gl/11 oz/1 large can mandarin oranges in syrup
60 ml/4 tbsp granulated sugar
5 ml/1 tsp finely grated orange peel
5 ml/1 tsp ginger jam (conserve)
90 ml/6 tbsp double (heavy) cream, whipped
Vanilla ice cream

Put the rhubarb in a 1.25 litre/2¼ pt/5½ cup dish with 30 ml/2 tbsp syrup from the mandarins and all the sugar. Cover with a plate and cook on Full for 7–9 minutes until the rhubarb is tender. Uncover and stir in the drained mandarins and orange peel. Cover and cool, then chill for several hours. Mix the jam lightly into the cream. Spoon the rhubarb and mandarin mixture into six glasses over scoops of ice cream and top each with 25 ml/1½ tbsp of the ginger cream. Eat straight away.

Chocolate Strawberries on Pineapple Sorbet

Serves 4

175 g/6 oz plain (semi-sweet) chocolate
15 g/½ oz/1 tbsp unsalted (sweet) butter
16–20 large unhulled strawberries, washed and dried
Pineapple sorbet

Break up the chocolate and place in a dish with the butter. Melt, uncovered, on Defrost for about 3½ minutes. If the chocolate stays on the firm side, give it 10-second bursts on Defrost until just runny – do not overheat or the chocolate will become granular. Holding each strawberry by its green hull and stalk, swirl it round in the chocolate until three-quarters covered. Stand on a baking tray lined with greaseproof (waxed) paper and leave in the cool to set. To serve, put scoops of sorbet into four glass dessert dishes and top each with the strawberries.

Danish Apple 'Cake'

Serves 4–6

An old friend from Denmark, and a distinguished and handsome-looking sundae – not remotely like a cake.

750 g/1½ lb cooking (tart) apples, peeled and sliced
45 ml/3 tbsp boiling water
90 ml/6 tbsp caster (superfine) sugar
125 g/4 oz/½ cup butter
100 g/3½ oz/1¾ cups fresh white breadcrumbs
30 ml/2 tbsp light soft brown sugar
150 ml/¼ pt/⅔ cup double (heavy) cream
15 ml/1 tbsp milk
20–60 ml/4–6 tsp red jam (conserve)

Put the apple slices in a 1.75 litre/3 pt/7½ cup dish with the boiling water. Cover with a plate and cook on Full for 7–8 minutes until very soft. Beat to a pulp, then stir in the caster sugar. Set aside. Melt the butter in a frying pan (skillet). Add the breadcrumbs and fry (sauté) conventionally until lightly browned. Stir in the brown sugar. Allow to cool. Fill four to six sundae or other tall glasses with alternate layers of apples and crumbs, ending with crumbs. Whip the cream and milk until softly stiff. Pile on top of each portion, then add 5 ml/1 tsp of jam to each.

Peasant Girl with Veil

Serves 4–6

A variation on Danish Apple Cake, this is also Danish but uses 5 slices of crumbled rye bread instead of white breadcrumbs. Otherwise the ingredients and method are the same.

Imperial Rice

Serves 6–8

An old French traditional recipe, simplified by the use of store cupboard ingredients.

400 g/14 oz/1 large can rice pudding
400–450 g/14–16 oz/1 large can custard
25 ml/1½ tbsp powdered gelatine
125 ml/4 fl oz/½ cup cold water
60 ml/4 tbsp smooth apricot jam (conserve)
5 ml/1 tsp vanilla essence (extract)
2.5 ml/½ tsp almond essence (extract)
30 ml/2 tbsp assorted coloured glacé (candied) cherries, coarsely chopped

Combine the rice pudding and custard in a 2 litre/3½ pt/8½ cup bowl. Put the gelatine into a small bowl and stir in half the water. Heat, uncovered, on Defrost for 1¾–2 minutes until melted and the liquid is clear. Add the remaining water. Stir gently into the rice and custard mixture. Spoon the jam into the emptied small bowl. Warm, uncovered, on Defrost for 1–1½ minutes. Stir into the rice mixture with the vanilla and almond essence (extract). Cover and chill until just on the point of setting. Stir in the cherries. Rinse a 1.5 litre/2½ pt/6 cup jelly (jello) mould with cold water, then fill with the rice mixture. Cover and chill until firm and set. Turn out and serve with any of the fruit sauces.

Children's Fruity Mousse

Serves 4–6

An easy and economical sweet that reached its heyday in the fifties.

1 packet strawberry jelly (jello)
300 ml/½ pt/1¼ cups cold water
175 ml/6 fl oz/1 small can full-cream evaporated milk, chilled overnight in the refrigerator
30 ml/2 tbsp fresh or bottled lemon juice
Whipped cream and fruit, to decorate (optional)

Snip the jelly into cubes and put in a measuring jug. Cover with a plate and melt on Defrost for 2–2½ minutes. Gradually stir in the water. Keep covered and leave in the cool until just beginning to thicken. Beat the chilled evaporated milk until light and frothy. Add the lemon juice, a little at a time, and continue whisking until the milk thickens to the consistency of whipped cream. Whisk in the still liquid jelly lightly but smoothly. Transfer to four to six small dishes and chill until set. Decorate with cream and/or canned or fresh fruit, if liked.

Raspberry and Blackcurrant Mousse

Serves 4

A more sophisticated version of Children's Fruity Mousse that can confidently be served to adults.

1 packet raspberry jelly (jello)
150 ml/¼ pt/2/3 cup cold water
150 ml/¼ pt/2/3 cup raspberry purée made from fresh or frozen raspberries
175 ml/6 fl oz/1 small can full-cream evaporated milk, chilled overnight in the refrigerator
30 ml/2 tbsp fresh or bottled lemon juice
Whipped cream and fresh blackcurrants, to decorate

Snip the jelly into cubes and put in a measuring jug. Cover with a plate and melt on Defrost for 2–2½ minutes. Gradually stir in the water and raspberry purée. Keep covered and leave in the cool until just beginning to thicken. Beat the chilled evaporated milk until light and frothy. Add the lemon juice, a little at a time, and continue whisking until the milk thickens to the consistency of whipped cream. Whisk in the still liquid jelly lightly but smoothly. Swirl into four wine glasses and chill until set. Decorate with cream and blackcurrants.

Welsh Rarebit

Serves 2

125 g/4 oz/1 cup Cheddar cheese, grated
5 ml/1 tsp mustard powder
5 ml/1 tsp cornflour (cornstarch)
1 egg yolk
10 ml/2 tsp milk
Salt and freshly ground black pepper
2 large slices freshly made toast
Paprika

Mix the cheese with the mustard, cornflour, egg yolk and milk. Season to taste. Spread over the toast. Transfer to individual plates. Cook one at a time, uncovered, on Full for 1 minute. Sprinkle lightly with paprika and eat straight away.

Mixed Cheese Rarebit

Serves 2

Prepare as for Welsh Rarebit, but substitute 50 g/2 oz/½ cup crumbled Stilton cheese for half the Cheddar.

Buck Rarebit

Serves 2

Prepare as for Welsh Rarebit, but top each slice with a fried (sautéed) egg, cooked either in the microwave or conventionally.

Bacon Rarebit

Serves 2

Put 4 streaky bacon rashers (slices) on a plate and cover with kitchen paper. Cook on Full for 2½ minutes. Prepare the Welsh Rarebit and top each slice with 2 bacon rashers.

Beer Rarebit

Serves 4

Slightly more ornate, this is a substantial snack for midday or the evening.

25 g/1 oz/2 tbsp butter or margarine, at kitchen temperature
5 ml/1 tsp mild made mustard
2.5 ml/½ tsp Worcestershire sauce
5 ml/1 tsp tomato ketchup (catsup)
225 g/8 oz/2 cups Cheddar cheese, grated
45 ml/3 tbsp dark ale
4 slices freshly made toast
1 large tomato, sliced
Chopped parsley
Bacon and fried (sautéed) or poached eggs (optional), to serve

Combine the butter or margarine with the mustard, Worcestershire sauce, ketchup, cheese and ale. Spread equal amounts over the toast. Transfer to four individual plates. Cook, uncovered one at a time, on Full for 1 minute. Add the tomato slices and a sprinkling of parsley. If liked, top with bacon and/or eggs.

Open-topped Hungarian Salami Sandwiches

Serves 4

These are based on a recipe found in a leaflet at a Hungarian trade fair held in London. The subtle smokiness of the salami gives the sandwiches a continental flair.

4 spring onions (scallions), finely chopped
75 g/3 oz Hungarian salami, rinded and finely chopped
175 g/6 oz/1½ cups Emmental cheese, finely grated
2 egg yolks
4 large slices freshly made toast
Pickled cucumber slices, to garnish

Put the onions and salami in a bowl and combine with the cheese and egg yolks. Spread over the toast. Cook one at a time, uncovered, on Full for 1–1½ minutes until the cheese melts. Serve straight away.

Granola

Makes about 750 g/1½ lb/6 cups

Like dry and sweet muesli with a distinctive crackle and a crunch, this is an import from North America where it is eaten as a breakfast cereal with milk or as a nibble instead of biscuits (cookies). Diet food it isn't, but it can be enjoyed as an occasional weekend treat.

125 g/4 oz/½ cup butter or margarine
90 ml/6 tbsp golden (light corn) syrup
250 g/9 oz/2¼ cups porridge oats
45 ml/3 tbsp coarse bran
100 g/3½ oz/scant ½ cup light soft brown sugar
75 g/3 oz/¾ cup chopped nuts
100 g/3½ oz/2/3 cup raisins

Put the butter or margarine in a 25 cm/10 in diameter casserole dish (Dutch oven). Add the syrup. Melt, uncovered, on Defrost for 4 minutes. Mix in all the remaining ingredients except the raisins. Cook, uncovered, on Full for 9½ minutes, stirring four or five times, until the granola is lightly browned. Add the raisins and mix in thoroughly. Allow to stand until cold and crisp, then break up with a fork until crumbly. Store in an airtight container.

Honey Granola

Makes about 750 g/1½ lb/6 cups

Prepare as for Granola, but substitute clear honey for the syrup.

Porridge

For 1 portion: put 25 g/1 oz/¼ cup porridge oats in a cereal bowl. Add 150 ml/¼ pt/2/3 cup cold milk or water and a pinch of salt. Cook, uncovered, on Full for 1¾–2 minutes, stirring twice. Allow to stand for 1½ minutes before eating.

For 2 portions in 2 bowls: prepare as for 1 portion, but cook on Full for 3–3½ minutes.

For 3 portions in 3 bowls: prepare as for 1 portion, but cook on Full for 3½ –4 minutes.

Bacon

Bacon reacts well to microwave cooking and shrinks less than if grilled (broiled) or fried (sautéed) conventionally. Place the rasher or rashers (slices) in a single layer on a plate and cover lightly with kitchen paper to prevent spluttering and soiling the oven. The cooking time needed will vary according to the type and thickness of the bacon, but this is a general guide:

1 rasher: cook on Full for 45–60 seconds

2 rashers: cook on Full for 1½–1¾ minutes

3 rashers: cook on Full for 2–2¼ minutes

4 rashers: cook on Full for 2½–2¾ minutes

5 rashers: cook on Full for 3–3½ minutes

6 rashers: cook on Full for 4–4½ minutes

Drain the bacon on clean kitchen paper after cooking.

Basic White Sauce

Serves 4

The multi-purpose and versatile coating sauce known and appreciated internationally for its smooth and velvety texture and glossy appearance.

300 ml/½ pt/1¼ cups milk
25 g/1 oz/2 tbsp butter or margarine
25 g/1 oz/¼ cup plain (all-purpose) flour
Salt and freshly ground black pepper or caster (superfine) sugar

Pour the milk into a jug and warm, uncovered, on Full for 2 minutes. Put the butter or margarine in a 900 ml/1½ pt/3¾ cup bowl. Melt, uncovered, on Defrost for 1 minute. Stir in the flour to form a roux. Heat, uncovered, on Full for 30 seconds. Remove from the microwave and gradually blend in the warm milk. Cook, uncovered, on Full for 3–4 minutes, beating every minute for maximum smoothness, until the sauce comes to the boil and thickens. Season to taste with salt and pepper for a savoury sauce and caster sugar for a sweet one.

Béchamel Sauce

Serves 4

This the aristocratic version of Basic White Sauce, named after a steward of Louis XIV. It is important in the great kitchens of the western world and is deceptively easy to make. Use only for savoury dishes.

300 ml/½ pt/1¼ cups milk
1 bouquet garni sachet
1 bay leaf
1 small onion, peeled and quartered
2 large parsley sprigs
1.5 ml/¼ tsp grated nutmeg
25 g/1 oz/2 tbsp butter or margarine
25 g/1 oz/¼ cup plain (all-purpose) flour
Salt and freshly ground black pepper

Pour the milk into a 900 ml/1½ pt/3¾ cup jug. Add the bouquet garni, bay leaf, onion, parsley and nutmeg. Cover with a saucer and bring just up to the boil, allowing 5–6 minutes on Defrost. Remove from the microwave, keep covered, and allow to cool to lukewarm. Strain. Put the butter or margarine in a 900 ml/1½ pt/3¾ cup bowl. Melt, uncovered, on Defrost for 1 minute. Stir in the flour to form a roux. Heat, uncovered, on Full for 30 seconds. Remove from the microwave and gradually blend in the flavoured milk. Cook, uncovered, on Full for 3–4 minutes, beating every minute for maximum smoothness, until the sauce comes to the boil and thickens. Season to taste with salt and pepper.

Caper Sauce

Serves 4

For skate, herring, mackerel and lamb.

Prepare as for Basic White Sauce, but add 20 ml/4 tsp drained and chopped capers half-way through the cooking time.

Cheese Sauce

Serves 4

For bacon and gammon, fish, poultry and vegetables.

Prepare as for Basic White Sauce, but add 50–75 g/2–3 oz/½–¾ cup grated hard cheese and 5 ml/1 tsp made mustard half-way through the cooking time.

Mornay Sauce

Serves 4

A close relation of Cheese Sauce, also for bacon and gammon, fish, poultry and vegetables.

Prepare as for Basic White Sauce, but use milk seasoned with salt and freshly ground black pepper and add 50–75 g/2–3 oz/½–¾ cup grated Gruyère (Swiss) cheese half-way through the cooking time.

Egg Sauce

Serves 4

Also known as Dutch Egg Sauce or Mock Hollandaise. For fish and poultry.

Prepare as for Basic White Sauce, but add 2 chopped hard-boiled (hard-cooked) eggs with the seasoning.

Mushroom Sauce

Serves 4

For fish and poultry and egg dishes such as omelettes.

Heat 50 g/2 oz/½ cup thinly sliced mushrooms with 10 ml/2 tsp butter on Full for 1½ minutes. Mix into the prepared Basic White Sauce half-way through the cooking time. Season to taste with ground nutmeg.

Mustard Sauce

Serves 4

Serve with pork and gammon, offal and oily fish such as mackerel and herring.

Prepare as for Basic White Sauce, but add 10–15 ml/2–3 tsp English made mustard and 10 ml/2 tsp lemon juice with the seasoning.

Onion Sauce

Serves 4

For grilled (broiled) and roast lamb.

Chop 1 onion and put into a small dish with 25 ml/1½ tbsp cold water and 1.5 ml/¼ tsp salt. Cover with clingfilm (plastic wrap) and slit it twice to allow steam to escape. Cook on Full for 4–5 minutes until soft. Mix into the prepared Basic White Sauce.

Parsley Sauce

Serves 4

For fish, vegetables, poultry and boiled bacon.

Prepare as for Basic White Sauce, but add 45–60 ml/3–4 tbsp chopped parsley with the seasoning.

Watercress Sauce

Serves 4

For fish and poultry.

Prepare as for Basic White Sauce, but add 45–60 ml/3–4 tbsp chopped watercress with the seasoning.

Pouring Sauce

Serves 4

Prepare as for Basic White Sauce, but reduce the flour to 15 g/½ oz/1 tbsp. Either season with salt and pepper and use as a white 'gravy', or sweeten with sugar and serve over steamed or baked pudding.

All-in-one Sauce

Serves 4

A high-speed version of Basic White Sauce.

25 g/1 oz/¼ cup plain (all-purpose) flour
300 ml/½ pt/1¼ cups milk
25 g/1 oz/2 tbsp butter or margarine
Salt and freshly ground black pepper or caster (superfine) sugar

Whisk the flour into the milk in a bowl, then add the butter or margarine. Cook, uncovered, on Full for 6–6½ minutes, whisking four or five times, until thick and smooth. Flavour to taste.

Hollandaise Sauce

Serves 6–8

One of the great sauces of our time, Hollandaise made conventionally needs skill and culinary artistry. In the microwave it behaves as though you were a chef of unquestionable brilliance. Use it with poached salmon and trout, broccoli and cauliflower, with artichokes and asparagus.

125 g/4 oz/½ cup slightly salted butter
15 ml/1 tbsp lemon juice, strained
2 egg yolks
Salt and freshly ground black pepper
A pinch of caster (superfine) sugar

Put the butter in a 900 ml/1½ pt/3¾ cup jug or dish. Melt, uncovered, on Full for 1½ minutes until hot and bubbling. Add the lemon juice and egg yolks and whisk thoroughly. Return to the microwave and cook on Full for 30 seconds. Stir briskly. The sauce is ready when it is as thick as cold custard and clings to the whisk; if not, cook for a further 15 seconds. Season to taste, then add the sugar to counteract the sharpness of the lemon juice. Serve warm. Watch the cooking time very carefully because Hollandaise that refuses to thicken and looks curdled has been overcooked. One remedy is to beat in 30–45 ml/2–3 tbsp very cold water; a second is to beat in 30 ml/2 tbsp double (heavy) cream; a third is to beat the curdled sauce into a fresh egg yolk and return to the microwave for a few seconds until thick and smooth.

Short-cut Béarnaise Sauce

Serves 6–8

Recommended for steaks and rare roast beef.

Prepare as for Hollandaise Sauce, but substitute wine vinegar for the lemon juice and add 2.5 ml/½ tsp dried tarragon with the seasoning and sugar.

Maltese Sauce

Serves 6–8

For freshwater fish and poultry.

Prepare as for Hollandaise Sauce, but stir in 5 ml/1 tsp very finely grated orange peel with the seasoning and sugar.

Mayonnaise Sauce

Makes 600 ml/1 pt/2½ cups

Because of the current disquiet associated with eating raw egg yolk, the eggs in this mayonnaise are blended with very hot liquid, which is equivalent to being partially cooked and is therefore safer than standard home-made mayonnaise based on entirely raw yolks. The texture is thinner than traditional mayonnaise but, when cold, is thick enough to coat foods satisfactorily. It is also excellent as a mixer sauce with coleslaw and potato salad.

600 ml/1 pt/2½ cups sunflower or safflower oil
30 ml/2 tbsp lemon juice
15 ml/1 tbsp wine or cider vinegar
2.5 ml/½ tsp caster (superfine) sugar
15–20 ml/3–4 tsp salt
5 ml/1 tsp made mustard
2 large eggs

Spoon 75 ml/5 tbsp of the oil into a small bowl. Add the lemon juice, vinegar, sugar, salt and mustard. Heat, uncovered, on Defrost for 3–4 minutes until very hot. Break the eggs into a blender and add the hot oil mixture. Run the machine until smooth. With the machine still running but the lid removed, add the remaining oil in a thin steady stream. Transfer to a bowl. Cover and chill until cold and thick. Keep refrigerated in screw-topped jar and use as required.

Cocktail Sauce

Makes 600 ml/1 pt/2½ cups

A classic for seafood.

Prepare as for Mayonnaise Sauce. After it has thickened, stir in 30 ml/2 tbsp tomato purée (paste), 10 ml/2 tsp horseradish, a dash of hot pepper sauce such as Tabasco and 5 ml/1 tsp Worcestershire sauce.

Louis Sauce

Makes 600 ml/1 pt/2½ cups

A sauce from San Francisco created in the early twentieth century by a chef called Louis Diat. It is specially for crab salad.

600 ml/1 pt/2½ cups sunflower or safflower oil
30 ml/2 tbsp lemon juice
15 ml/1 tbsp wine or cider vinegar
2.5 ml/½ tsp caster (superfine) sugar
15–20 ml/3–4 tsp salt
5 ml/1 tsp made mustard
2 large eggs
Chilli or hot pepper sauce
60 ml/4 tbsp whipping cream, softly whipped
¼ green (bell) pepper, seeded and finely chopped
15 ml/1 tbsp finely chopped spring onion (scallion)
Juice of ½ small lemon

Spoon 75 ml/5 tbsp of the oil into a small bowl. Add the lemon juice, vinegar, sugar, salt and mustard. Heat, uncovered, on Defrost for 3–4 minutes until very hot. Break the eggs into a blender and add the hot oil mixture. Run the machine until smooth. With the machine still running but the lid removed, add the remaining oil in a thin steady stream. Transfer to a bowl. Cover and chill until cold and thick. Stir in chilli or hot pepper sauce to make it gently hot, then add the cream, green pepper, spring onion and lemon juice. Keep refrigerated in a screw-topped jar and use as required.

Thousand Island Dressing

Makes 600 ml/1 pt/2½ cups

600 ml/1 pt/2½ cups sunflower or safflower oil
30 ml/2 tbsp lemon juice
15 ml/1 tbsp wine or cider vinegar
2.5 ml/½ tsp caster (superfine) sugar
15–20 ml/3–4 tsp salt
5 ml/1 tsp made mustard
2 large eggs
A dash of chilli or hot pepper sauce
1–2 hard-boiled (hard-cooked) eggs (pages 98–9), finely chopped
30–45 ml/2–3 tbsp tomato ketchup (catsup)
15 ml/1 tbsp finely chopped onion
15 ml/1 tbsp chopped parsley
30 ml/2 tbsp chopped stuffed olives (optional)
30 ml/2 tbsp whipped cream (optional)

Spoon 75 ml/5 tbsp of the oil into a small bowl. Add the lemon juice, vinegar, sugar, salt and mustard. Heat, uncovered, on Defrost for 3–4 minutes until very hot. Break the eggs into a blender and add the hot oil mixture. Run the machine until smooth. With the machine still running but the lid removed, add the remaining oil in a thin steady stream. Transfer to a bowl. Cover and chill until cold and thick. Stir in the chilli or hot pepper sauce, chopped eggs, tomato ketchup, onion, parsley and olives and cream, if using. Keep refrigerated in a screw-topped jar and use as required.

Green Sauce

Makes 600 ml/1 pt/2½ cups

Designed for fish.

Prepare as for Mayonnaise Sauce. After it has thickened, stir in 15 ml/1 tbsp chopped parsley, 15 ml/1 tbsp snipped chives and 15 ml/1 tbsp watercress. A little chopped tarragon may also be added.

Rémoulade Sauce

Makes 600 ml/1 pt/2½ cups

Superb with cold meats, beef in particular, and fish dishes.

Prepare as for Mayonnaise Sauce. After it has thickened, mix in 4 chopped anchovy fillets in oil, 5 ml/1 tsp French mustard, 5 ml/1 tsp chopped tarragon and 5 ml/1 tsp chopped parsley, 10 ml/2 tsp chopped gherkins (cornichons) and 10 ml/2 tsp chopped capers. A little chopped chervil may also be added.

Sauce Tartare

Makes 600 ml/1 pt/2½ cups

For fish.

Prepare as for Mayonnaise Sauce. After it has thickened, stir in 45 ml/3 tbsp chopped gherkins (cornichons), 30 ml/2 tbsp chopped parsley and 15 ml/1 tbsp finely chopped capers.

No-egg Mayonnaise-style Dressing

Serves 4

60 ml/4 tbsp cold water
90 ml/6 tbsp sunflower oil
1 oz/25 g/1/3 cup milk powder (non-fat dry milk)
2.5 ml/½ tsp salt
2.5 ml/½ tsp mustard powder
20 ml/4 tsp wine or cider vinegar
10 ml/2 tsp lemon juice
A pinch of sugar

Pour the water into a small bowl. Heat, uncovered, on Full for 1 minute until hot. Pour into blender or food processor and add all the remaining ingredients. Run the machine until smooth. Spoon into small bowl, cover and chill until cold. The dressing thickens up considerably if left overnight but can be thinned down to the desired consistency with warm water.

Mint Sauce

Serves 4–5

A very British sauce for roast lamb.
60 ml/4 tbsp finely chopped fresh mint leaves
60 ml/4 tbsp water
15 ml/1 tbsp caster (superfine) sugar
75 ml/5 tbsp malt vinegar
Salt and freshly ground black pepper

Put all the ingredients into a measuring cup. Heat, uncovered, on Full for 3 minutes. Serve cold.

Orange Sauce

serves 6–8

For cold meats and barbecued foods.
225 g/8 oz/1 cup redcurrant jelly (clear conserve)
Finely grated peel and juice of 1 orange
10 ml/2 tsp Grand Marnier

Put the redcurrant jelly with the orange peel and juice in a 1.25 litre/2¼ pt/5½ cup measuring jug. Heat, uncovered, on Defrost for 5–6 minutes, stirring three or four times, until the jelly melts. Allow the sauce to cool, then mix in the Grand Marnier. Serve cold.

Jellied Mixed Herb Sauce

Serves 8–10

For lamb.

450 ml/¾ pt/2 cups white grape or apple juice
15 ml/1 tbsp powdered gelatine
2.5 ml/½ tsp salt
30 ml/2 tbsp chopped mint
45 ml/3 tbsp snipped chives
40 ml/2½ tbsp chopped coriander (cilantro) leaves

Pour 45 ml/3 tbsp of the fruit juice into a 1.25 litre/2¼ pt/5½ cup bowl. Stir in the gelatine. Allow to stand for 5 minutes to soften. Melt, uncovered, on Defrost for 2–2½ minutes. Stir in the remaining juice with the salt. Cover when cold and chill until just beginning to thicken and set round the edge. Mix in all the remaining ingredients. Transfer to a small serving dish and chill until set completely. Spoon out on to plates to serve.

Jellied Herb Sauce with Lemon

Serves 8–10

For fish.

Prepare as for Jellied Mixed Herb Sauce, but substitute chopped parsley for the coriander (cilantro) and add 10 ml/2 tsp grated lemon rind with the other ingredients.

Salsa

Serves 6

A simple version of the trendy Mexican sauce-cum-condiment which can be used as a dip or eaten with Mexican-style food. It also adds a bit of character to roasts and grilled (broiled) foods, bland cheeses like Mozzarella and omelettes. Some salsas are left uncooked, but heating this rather chunky version has a mellowing effect on the flavours.

3 large tomatoes, blanched, skinned, seeded and chopped
1 sweet or Spanish onion, finely grated
1–2 whole green chillies, seeded and finely chopped
1–2 garlic cloves, crushed
30 ml/2 tbsp chopped coriander (cilantro) leaves
5–10 ml/1–2 tsp salt

Place the tomatoes in a 1.25 litre/2¼ pt/5½ cup bowl with the onion, chilli and garlic. Cover with a plate and heat on Full for 3 minutes. Allow to cool completely. Stir in the coriander and salt before serving.

Smooth Salsa

Serves 6

Prepare as for Salsa, but transfer the ingredients to a blender after cooking and work to a smooth purée before adding the coriander and salt.

Extra-hot Salsa

Serves 6

Prepare as for Salsa, but double or even treble the quantity of green chillies. Take care when eating.

Coriander Salsa

Serves 6

Prepare as for Salsa, but increase the quantity of coriander (cilantro) to 25 g/1 oz/¼ cup.

Apple Sauce

Serves 4

Obligatory for roast pork, duck and goose.

450 g/1 lb cooking (tart) apples, peeled, quartered, cored and thinly sliced
45 ml/3 tbsp boiling water
10–15 ml/2–3 tsp granulated sugar
10 ml/2 tsp butter or margarine

Put the apples in a 1.25 litre/2¼ pt/5½ cup bowl with the water. Cover with a plate and cook on Full for 7–8 minutes until soft and pulpy, stirring twice. Beat until smooth. Mix in the sugar and butter or margarine. Serve warm or cold.

Mrs Beeton's Brown Apple Sauce

Serves 4

Prepare as for Apple Sauce, but cook the apples with a thin gravy instead of water.

Gooseberry Sauce

Serves 4

An old English sauce, traditionally served with goose, duck and mackerel.

Prepare as for Apple Sauce, but substitute 225 g/8 oz/2 cups trimmed gooseberries for the apples and add 5 ml/1 tsp finely grated lemon peel with the other ingredients.

Salsa with Sweetcorn

Serves 4

For barbecued foods.

10 ml/2 tsp corn oil
3 spring onions (scallions), finely chopped
30 ml/2 tbsp finely chopped coriander (cilantro) leaves
1 canned red pimiento, drained and chopped
2 large beef tomatoes, blanched, skinned, seeded and chopped
175 g/6 oz/1½ cups frozen sweetcorn (corn), thawed
10 ml/2 tsp jalapeno sauce
10 ml/2 tsp fresh lime juice
5 ml/1 tsp salt

Pour the oil into a 1.25 litre/2¼ pt/5½ cup bowl. Add the onions, coriander and pimiento. Cook, uncovered, on Full for 2½ minutes, stirring once. Mix in the tomatoes and sweetcorn. Cover with a plate and heat on Full for 2 minutes. Allow to cool completely. Stir in the remaining ingredients.

Austrian Apple and Horseradish Sauce

Serves 6–8

An example of the unusual and the unexpected, a remarkable hot sauce for beef.

450 g/1 lb cooking (tart) apples, peeled, quartered, cored and thinly sliced
30 ml/2 tbsp boiling water
10 ml/2 tsp icing (confectioners') sugar, sifted
30 ml/2 tbsp blanched and finely chopped almonds
15–45 ml/1–3 tbsp finely grated fresh horseradish or 30–45 ml/2–3 tbsp creamed horseradish
2.5–5 ml/½–1 tsp salt
10 ml/2 tsp malt vinegar

Put the apples in a 1.25 litre/2¼ pt/5½ cup bowl with the water. Cover with a plate and cook on Full for 7–8 minutes until soft and pulpy, stirring twice. Stir in all the remaining ingredients. Cover as before and cook on Full for 1½ minutes. Serve hot.

Garlic Sauce

Serves 4–6

An extremely garlicky sauce from Italy, designed for tossing into hot pasta dishes.

45 ml/3 tbsp olive oil

50 g/2 oz/¼ cup butter

6 garlic cloves, crushed

30 ml/2 tbsp finely chopped parsley

2.5 ml/½ tsp dried basil

2.5–5 ml/½–1 tsp salt

Freshly ground black pepper, to taste

Put all the ingredients in a 600 ml/1 pt/2½ cup bowl. Cover with a plate and warm on Defrost for 3–4 minutes, stirring once. Toss with piping hot spaghetti or other pasta and eat straight away.

Apple and Horseradish Sauce

Serves 6–8

An apple sauce from Romania, to serve with chicken.

50 g/2 oz/¼ cup butter
2 large cooking (tart) apples, peeled and grated
50 g/2 oz/½ cup plain (all-purpose) flour
450 ml/¾ pt/2 cups hot chicken stock
5–10 ml/1–2 tsp grated horseradish or 10 ml/2 tsp horseradish sauce
Salt
150 ml/¼ pt/2/3 cup whipping cream, whipped until thick
Sifted icing (confectioners') sugar (optional)

Put the butter in a 1.5 litre/2½ pt/6 cup bowl and heat, uncovered, on Full for 1¼ minutes. Mix in the apples and cook, uncovered, on Full for 3 minutes, stirring once. Stir in the flour and cook on Full for 20 seconds. Gradually blend in the hot stock. Cook, uncovered, on Full for 4–5 minutes, whisking every minute, until smoothly thickened. Stir in the horseradish, season to taste with salt, then fold in the cream. If the sauce is too sour for personal taste, stir in a little icing sugar. Serve straight away.

Bread Sauce

Serves 6–8

A vintage tradition with poultry.

300 ml/½ pt/1¼ cups milk

1 bouquet garni sachet

1 bay leaf

1 small onion, peeled and quartered

2 large parsley sprigs

1.5 ml/¼ tsp grated nutmeg

65 g/2½ oz fresh white breadcrumbs from crustless bread

15–25 g/½–1 oz/1–2 tbsp butter or margarine

Salt and freshly ground black pepper

Pour the milk into a 900 ml/1½ pt/3¾ cup jug. Add the bouquet garni, bay leaf, onion, parsley and nutmeg. Cover with a saucer and bring just to the boil on Defrost, allowing about 5–6 minutes. Remove from the microwave, keep covered and allow to cool to lukewarm. Strain. Add the crumbs. Cook, uncovered, on Defrost until thickened, allowing about 4–6 minutes and stirring every minute. Mix in the butter or margarine and season to taste. Reheat, uncovered, on Defrost for 1 minute.

Brown Bread Sauce

Serves 6–8

Prepare as for Bread Sauce, but substitute fresh breadcrumbs from crustless brown bread in place of the white.

Cranberry Sauce

Serves 6–8

A sweet-sour, fruity winter sauce and a sparkling and brilliant accompaniment for poultry.

225 g/8 oz/2 cups cranberries, thawed if frozen
150 ml/¼ pt/⅔ cup water
175 g/6 oz/¾ cup granulated sugar
5 ml/1 tsp finely grated lemon peel

Put all the ingredients in a 1.25 litre/2¼ pt/5½ cup bowl. Cover with a plate and cook on Full for 8–8½ minutes, stirring twice and crushing the fruit against the side of the bowl, until the fruit is soft. Remove from the microwave, keep covered and serve when cold. Keep any leftovers refrigerated in a covered container.

Cranberry Wine Sauce

Serves 6–8

Prepare as for Cranberry Sauce, but substitute red wine for the water.

Cranberry Orange Sauce

Serves 6–8

Prepare as for Cranberry Sauce, but substitute orange juice for the water.

Cranberry and Apple Sauce

Serves 6–8

Prepare as for Cranberry Sauce, but substitute 1 sliced cooking (tart) apple for half the cranberries.

Cumberland Sauce

Serves 6

A full-bodied and typically English sauce for ham, pork and tongue.

5 ml/1 tsp mild made mustard

30 ml/2 tbsp light soft brown sugar

1.5 ml/¼ tsp ground ginger

A pinch of cayenne pepper

300 ml/½ pt/1¼ cups dry white wine or port

2 whole cloves

15 ml/1 tbsp cornflour (cornstarch)

30 ml/2 tbsp cold water

60 ml/4 tbsp redcurrant jelly (clear conserve)

5 ml/1 tsp grated orange peel

5 ml/1 tsp grated lemon peel

Juice of 1 small orange

Juice of 1 lemon

Put the mustard, sugar, ginger, cayenne, wine or port and cloves in a 1.25 litre/2¼ pt/5½ cup bowl and heat, uncovered, on Full for 6 minutes, stirring three times. Meanwhile, mix the cornflour smoothly with the cold water. Mix into the wine mixture with the remaining ingredients. Heat, uncovered, on Full for 4–6 minutes, stirring every minute, until the sauce is thickened and smooth and the jelly has melted. Serve hot.

Slovenian Wine Sauce

Serves 4–6

A vegetable purée and wine sauce enriched with cream. It goes particularly well with venison and pigeon.

50 g/2 oz/¼ cup salted butter
2 carrots, finely grated
30 ml/2 tbsp plain (all-purpose) flour
300 ml/½ pt/1¼ cups dry white wine
100 g/3½ oz mushrooms, sliced
1 small bay leaf
Salt and freshly ground black pepper
150 ml/¼ pt/2/3 cup soured (dairy sour) cream

Put the butter in a 1.25 litre/2¼ pt/5½ cup bowl and heat, uncovered, on Full for 1¼ minutes. Add the carrots. Two-thirds cover with a plate and cook on Full for 4 minutes, stirring twice. Mix in the flour, wine, mushrooms and bay leaf. Cover with a plate and cook on Full for 6–7 minutes until the ingredients are tender. Remove the bay leaf and season to taste. Transfer to a blender or food processor and work to a smooth purée. Return to the dish and stir in the cream. Reheat on Full for 1–1½ minutes.

Thin Gravy for Poultry

Serves 6

15 ml/1 tbsp cornflour (cornstarch)
25 ml/1½ tbsp cold water
1 chicken or vegetable stock cube or 7.5 ml/1½ tsp brown gravy powder
300 ml/½ pt/1¼ cups stock, including pan juices from a roast chicken or turkey
Salt and freshly ground black pepper

Blend the cornflour smoothly with the cold water in a 900 ml/1½ pt/3¾ cup bowl or jug. Crumble in the stock cube or mix in the gravy powder. Stir in the stock. Cook, uncovered, on Full for 4–6 minutes, stirring every minute, until the gravy has thickened slightly. Season to taste before serving.

Thick Gravy for Meat

Serves 6

Prepare as for Thin Gravy for Poultry, but use 30 ml/2 tbsp cornflour (cornstarch) mixed with 40 ml/2½ tbsp cold water.

Short-cut Oriental Sauce

Serves 6–8

A cross between an Indian and a Malaysian sauce, this is a marvellous vehicle for adding flavour to leftover cold meat and sausages.

300 ml/10 fl oz/1 can condensed cream of celery or mushroom soup

150 ml/¼ pt/2/3 cup boiling water

30 ml/2 tbsp tomato purée (paste)

15 ml/1 tbsp mild or hot curry paste

1 garlic clove, crushed

5 ml/1 tsp turmeric

30 ml/2 tbsp fruit chutney

15 ml/1 tbsp crunchy peanut butter

20 ml/4 tsp desiccated (shredded) coconut

Pour the soup into a 1.25 litre/2¼ pt/5½ cup bowl with half the water. Add all the remaining ingredients except the coconut. Cover with a plate and heat on Full for 4 minutes, whisking every minute. Allow to stand for 2 minutes. Whisk in the remaining water and the coconut. Reheat, uncovered on Full for 1 minute.

Indonesian-style Peanut Sauce

Serves 6–8

In the Far East this sauce is served over assorted cold cooked vegetables, rather like a salad dressing, but it can also be used as a punchy sauce for barbecued foods and meat on skewers.

15 ml/1 tbsp corn oil
2 onions, finely chopped
1 garlic clove, crushed
350 g/12 oz/1½ cups smooth peanut butter
10 ml/2 tsp light soft brown sugar
Juice of 1 small lemon
600 ml/1 pt/2½ cups boiling water
30 ml/2 tbsp brown table sauce
Salt and freshly ground black pepper

Pour the oil into a 1.25 litre/2¼ pt/5½ cup bowl. Heat on Full for 30 seconds. Stir in the onions and garlic. Cook, uncovered, on Full for 6 minutes, stirring three times. Mix in the peanut butter, sugar, lemon juice and half the water. Cook, uncovered, on Full for 2–3 minutes, stirring three times, until the sauce looks like porridge in texture. Remove from the microwave. Thin down the sauce by whisking in the remaining water, then season with the brown sauce and salt and pepper to taste.

Creole Sauce

Serves 6–8

A jazzy sauce from the Mississippi, featuring sunset colours and an abundance of Mediterranean produce. It goes well with eggs, poultry, beef and even makes a vegetarian topping for fluffy mashed potatoes or rice.

20 ml/4 tsp corn oil
1 large onion, grated
1 garlic clove, crushed
30 ml/2 tbsp stoned (pitted) green olives, chopped
½ small green (bell) pepper, seeded and finely chopped
50 g/2 oz mushrooms, chopped
1 small bay leaf
400 g/14 oz/1 large can chopped tomatoes
15 ml/1 tbsp chopped basil leaves
15 ml/1 tbsp chopped parsley
10 ml/2 tsp dark soft brown sugar
5 ml/1 tsp salt
5 ml/1 tsp Tabasco or any other hot pepper sauce
5 cm/2 inch strip lemon peel

Put the oil, onion and garlic in a 2 litre/3½ pt/8½ cup bowl. Cook, uncovered, on Full for 6 minutes, stirring three times. Mix in the olives, green pepper and mushrooms. Cook, uncovered, on Full for 2 minutes. Stir in all the remaining ingredients. Cover with clingfilm (plastic wrap) and slit it twice to allow steam to escape. Cook on Full for 6–7 minutes, turning the bowl three times, until the sauce is hot. Allow to stand for 2 minutes before using.

Quick Creole Sauce

Serves 4–6

30 ml/2 tbsp dried (bell) pepper flakes
300 ml/10 fl oz/1 can condensed tomato soup
75 ml/5 tbsp boiling water
2.5 ml/½ tsp dried oregano
5 ml/1 tsp light soft brown sugar
5 ml/1 tsp Worcestershire sauce

Cover the pepper flakes with boiling water and leave for 3 minutes. Drain thoroughly. Put the soup and measured boiling water in a 1.25 litre/2¼ pt/5½ cup dish and beat until smooth. Mix in the remaining ingredients. Heat, uncovered, on Full for 4–5 minutes, stirring three times, until very hot.

Newburg Sauce

Serves 4

Associated primarily with lobster, this grandiose sauce goes equally well with many other shellfish, crab in particular.

25 g/1 oz/2 tbsp butter
1 small onion, grated
30 ml/2 tbsp plain (all-purpose) flour
300 ml/½ pt/1¼ cups single (light) cream, heated to lukewarm
3 egg yolks
60 ml/4 tbsp dry sherry or white port
Salt and freshly ground black pepper

Melt the butter, uncovered, on Full for 1 minute in a 900 ml/1½ pt/3¾ cup bowl. Add the onion and cook, uncovered, on Full for 1 minute, stirring once. Stir in the flour and cook, uncovered, on Full for 1 minute. Gradually blend in the cream. Cook, uncovered, on Full for 4–4½ minutes, whisking every minute, until thickened and smooth. Beat together the egg yolks and sherry or port. Add to the sauce and season to taste. Return to the microwave and cook, uncovered, on Defrost for 1–1½ minutes. Whisk and serve.

Piquant Brown Sauce

Serves 4–6

Based on a classic French sauce, this is a cheat's version that turns up trumps for grilled (broiled) foods and roasts and old family friends like sausages, toad-in-the-hole and corned beef.

300 ml/10 fl oz/1 can condensed oxtail soup
75 ml/5 tbsp boiling water
15 ml/1 tbsp chopped coriander (cilantro) leaves
15 ml/1 tbsp chopped parsley
15 ml/1 tbsp chopped capers
15 ml/1 tbsp chopped gherkins (cornichons)
2.5 ml/½ tsp dried mixed herbs
15 ml/1 tbsp brown table sauce
15 ml/1 tbsp port
Salt and freshly ground black pepper

Put all the ingredients in a 1.25 litre/2¼ pt/5½ cup bowl and heat, uncovered, on Full for 5 minutes, whisking every minute, until hot and smooth.

Piquant Sauce with Pickled Walnuts

Serves 4–6

Prepare as for Piquant Brown Sauce, but substitute 15 ml/1 tbsp chopped pickled walnuts for the capers.

Portuguese Sauce

Serves 6

The lovely flavour of this fresh tomato sauce does wondrous things to salmon and also cheers up roasted chicken and turkey.

30 ml/2 tbsp olive oil
1 onion, finely grated
2 rashers (slices) streaky bacon, finely chopped
1–2 garlic cloves, crushed
1 small carrot, grated
30 ml/2 tbsp plain (all-purpose) flour
5 tomatoes, blanched, skinned and chopped
45 ml/3 tbsp tomato purée (paste)
150 ml/¼ pt/2/3 cup boiling meat or vegetable stock
10 ml/2 tsp pickling spice, tied in a piece of muslin
10 ml/2 tsp dark soft brown sugar
5 ml/1 tsp salt
5 cm/2 in strip lemon peel
10 ml/2 tsp fresh lemon juice
Freshly ground black pepper

Put the oil, onion, bacon, garlic and carrot in a 2 litre/3½ pt/8½ cup bowl. Cook, uncovered, on Full for 4 minutes, stirring twice. Mix in the flour and cook on Full for 1 minute. Stir in all the remaining ingredients, adding pepper to taste. Cover with clingfilm (plastic wrap) and slit it twice to allow steam to escape. Cook on full for 7 minutes, turning twice. Allow to stand for 3 minutes. Strain into a clean dish. Cover with a plate and reheat on Full for 2–3 minutes before serving.

Rustic Tomato Sauce

Serves 4–6

30 ml/2 tbsp olive oil
1 onion, very finely chopped
2 celery stalks, finely chopped
1 rasher (slice) streaky bacon, finely chopped
1 small carrot, grated
1 garlic clove, crushed
25 ml/1½ tbsp plain (all-purpose) flour
400 g/14 oz/1 large can plum tomatoes, mashed
30 ml/2 tbsp tomato purée (paste)
10 ml/2 tsp dark soft brown sugar
1.5 ml/¼ tsp grated nutmeg
2.5 ml/½ tsp salt
150 ml/¼ pt/2/3 cup boiling stock or water

Put the oil in a 2 litre/3½ pt/8½ cup bowl. Mix in the onion, celery, bacon, carrot and garlic. Cook, uncovered, on Full for 4½ minutes, stirring twice. Mix in the flour. Cook, uncovered, on Full for 30 seconds. Add all the remaining ingredients and stir thoroughly to mix. Part-cover with a plate and cook on Full for 7 minutes, stirring three times. Allow to stand for 2 minutes.

Curried Turkey Sauce for Jacket Potatoes

Serves 6

15 ml/1 tbsp corn oil
2 onions, chopped
20 ml/4 tsp mild, medium or hot curry powder
350 g/12 oz/3 cups minced (ground) turkey
20 ml/4 tsp plain flour
150 ml/¼ pt/2/3 cup canned coconut milk
150 ml/¼ pt/2/3 cup water
30 ml/2 tbsp tomato purée (paste)
15 ml/1 tbsp fruit chutney
5 ml/1 tsp salt
Juice of 1 lime
30 ml/2 tbsp apple juice
150 ml/¼ pt/2/3 cup thick plain yoghurt

Pour the oil into a 1.25 litre/2¼ pt/5½ cup bowl. Heat on Full for 30 seconds. Mix in the onions and curry powder. Cook, uncovered, on Full for 5 minutes, stirring three times. Stir in the turkey. Cover with a plate and cook on Full for 6 minutes, stirring with a fork three or four times to keep the turkey crumbly. Mix in all the remaining ingredients except the yoghurt. Cover as before and cook on Full for 4 minutes, stirring twice. Allow to stand for 4 minutes. Spoon into split jacket potatoes and top each with a dollop of thick yoghurt.

Tandoori Turkey Sauce for Jacket Potatoes

Serves 6

Prepare as for Curried Turkey Sauce for Jacket Potatoes, but substitute tandoori powder for curry powder.

Hot Chilli Beef Sauce for Jacket Potatoes

Serves 6

60 ml/4 tbsp corn or sunflower oil
2 onions, chopped
2 cloves garlic, crushed
350 g/12 oz/3 cups lean minced (ground) beef
30 ml/2 tbsp plain (all-purpose) flour
2.5–10 ml/½–2 tsp chilli powder
30 ml/2 tbsp tomato purée (paste)
300 ml/½ pt/1¼ cups hot water
5 ml/1 tsp salt
45 ml/3 tbsp dry cider

Pour the oil into a 1.25 litre/2¼ pt/5½ cup dish. Mix in the onions and garlic. Cook, uncovered, on Full for 5 minutes, stirring twice. Stir in the beef. Cover with a plate and cook on Full for 6 minutes, stirring with a fork three or four times to keep the meat crumbly. Stir in the remaining ingredients. Cover with clingfilm (plastic wrap) and slit it twice to allow steam to escape. Cook on Full for 6 minutes, turning the dish twice, until bubbling. Allow to stand for 5 minutes. Stir round, then spoon into split jacket potatoes.

Chop House Sauce

Serves 4

An assertive sauce from Edwardian days for grilled chops, chicken and steaks. A little goes a long way, which is why the quantities are small.

15 ml/1 tbsp tomato ketchup (catsup)
5–10 ml/1–2 tsp anchovy essence (extract)
5 ml/1 tsp English made mustard
15 ml/1 tbsp wine vinegar
45 ml/3 tbsp double (heavy) cream
2.5 ml/½ tsp Worcestershire sauce
A dash of hot pepper sauce

Put all the ingredients in a 600 ml/1 pt/2½ cup measuring jug. Warm through, uncovered, on Full for 1¼ –1½ minutes, stirring twice, until hot but not boiling. Use straight away.

Hot Cheese and Carrot Sauce for Jacket Potatoes

Serves 4

A vegetarian sauce with a zippy temperament.

25 g/1 oz/2 tbsp butter or margarine
1 large carrot, grated
30 ml/2 tbsp plain (all-purpose) flour
300 ml/½ pt/1¼ cups warmed milk
5 ml/1 tsp mustard powder
1.5 ml/¼ tsp cayenne pepper
A pinch of ground nutmeg
2.5 ml/½ tsp salt
2.5 ml/½ tsp dried marjoram
50 g/2 oz/½ cup grated cheese

Put the butter or margarine in a 1.25 litre/2¼ pt/5½ cup dish. Melt, uncovered, on Defrost for 1 minute. Stir in the carrot. Cook, uncovered, on Full for 4 minutes, stirring twice. Mix in the flour. Cook, uncovered, on Full for 30 seconds, then gradually blend in the warmed milk. Cook, uncovered, on Full for 4 minutes, stirring vigorously every minute. Stir in the remaining ingredients. Cook on Full for 30 seconds. Stir round and spoon into split jacket potatoes.

Basting Sauces

Brushed over meat joints, poultry and foods on the barbecue, bastes increase browning and make them look more appetising. They also add to the flavour and can be used as a basis for gravy and savoury sauces.

Butter Baste

Makes about 60 ml/4 tbsp

25 g/1 oz/2 tbsp butter or margarine, at kitchen temperature
15 ml/1 tbsp tomato purée (paste)
5 ml/1 tsp paprika
5 ml/1 tsp Worcestershire sauce
5 ml/1 tsp light soft brown sugar

Melt the butter, uncovered, on Defrost for 1–1½ minutes. Stir in the remaining ingredients. Reheat on Defrost for 30 seconds and use as required.

Spicy Curry Baste

Makes about 60 ml/4 tbsp

Prepare as for Butter Baste, but stir in 5 ml/1 tsp mild curry powder, 5 ml/1 tsp mustard powder, 2.5 ml/½ tsp garlic salt and a pinch of turmeric with the remaining ingredients.

Jalapeno Mexican Barbecue Baste

Serves 6

You can't mistake the south-of-the-border kick from this one, which perks up barbecued pork and chicken like nothing else.

150 ml/¼ pt/2/3 cup French dressing
45 ml/3 tbsp tomato ketchup (catsup)
15 ml/1 tbsp soy sauce
15 ml/1 tbsp Worcestershire sauce
15 ml/1 tbsp jalapeno sauce
15 ml/1 tbsp fresh lime juice
2.5 ml/½ tsp dried mixed herbs

Put all the ingredients in a 600 ml/1 pt/2½ cup dish. Cover with a saucer and heat on Full for 2½ minutes. Stir round and use for basting.

Tomato Baste

Makes about 60 ml/4 tbsp

A non-fat baste, ideal for slimmers and those on low-fat diets and also with rich meats such as pork, duck and goose.

15 ml/1 tbsp tomato purée (paste)
5 ml/1 tsp English made mustard
5 ml/1 tsp malt vinegar
5 ml/1 tsp Worcestershire sauce

Thoroughly mix together all the ingredients in a jug and heat, uncovered, on Full for 10 seconds.

Dutch Butter Blender Cream

Serves 4–6

Lush to eat and a cream that can be made when you run out of fresh or fancy something a bit different. It can be whipped to peaks like whipping cream and melts over hot food like ice cream.

150 ml/¼ pt/2/3 cup full-cream milk
150 g/5 oz/2/3 cup Dutch unsalted (sweet) butter

Pour the milk into a bowl. Cut in the pieces of butter. Heat, uncovered on Full for 2½ minutes. Transfer carefully to a blender and run the machine for 1 minute. Return to the washed and dried bowl, cover and chill for 2–3 hours. Spoon over puddings or whip softly, if preferred.

Dutch Butter Blender Cream with Vanilla

Serves 4–6

Prepare as for Dutch Butter Blender Cream, but add 5 ml/1 tsp vanilla essence (extract) to the milk and butter in the blender.

Hot Chocolate Sauce

Serves 6

An old classic for ice cream, ice cream sundaes and profiteroles.

25 g/1 oz/2 tbsp butter
30 ml/2 tbsp light soft brown sugar
30 ml/2 tbsp cocoa (unsweetened chocolate) powder
30 ml/2 tbsp golden (light corn) syrup
30 ml/2 tbsp single (light) cream
5 ml/1 tsp vanilla essence (extract)

Put the butter in a 600 ml/1 pt/2½ cup dish. Melt, uncovered, on Full for 1 minute. Thoroughly stir in all the remaining ingredients. Cook, uncovered, on Defrost for 5 minutes, stirring every minute, until the sauce is smooth and hot.

Mocha Sauce

Serves 6

Prepare as for Hot Chocolate Sauce, but add 20 ml/4 tsp instant coffee powder or granules before heating.

Hot Chocolate and Orange Sauce

Serves 6

Prepare as for Hot Chocolate Sauce, but stir in 10 ml/2 tsp finely grated orange peel after cooking.

Hot Chocolate Peppermint Sauce

Serves 6

Prepare as for Hot Chocolate sauce, but add a few drops of peppermint essence (extract) after cooking.

Raspberry Coulis

Serves 6–8

A clear – almost glassy – brilliant red sauce beloved by chefs for its stunning effect.

350 g/12 oz/3 cups fresh raspberries
45 ml/3 tbsp caster (superfine) sugar
15 ml/1 tbsp cornflour (cornstarch)
75 ml/5 tbsp cold water
5 ml/1 tsp vanilla essence (extract)
5 ml/1 tsp lemon juice

Carefully rinse the raspberries, then put in a food processor or blender and work to a purée. Strain through fine-mesh sieve (strainer) to remove the seeds. Transfer to a 900 ml/1½ pt/3¾ cup bowl with the sugar. Mix the cornflour smoothly with the water. Add to the purée in the bowl. Cook, uncovered, on Full for 2½–3½ minutes, whisking every 30 seconds, until the mixture has thickened and is clear and bubbling gently. Stir in the vanilla and lemon juice and use cold.

Summer Fruit Coulis

Serves 6–8

Prepare as for Raspberry Coulis, but substitute a mixture of summer fruits for the raspberries.

Apricot Coulis

Serves 6–8

450 g/1 lb stoned (pitted) apricots
200 ml/7 fl oz/scant 1 cup cold water
60–75 ml/4–5 tbsp caster (superfine) sugar
15 ml/1 tbsp cornflour (cornstarch)
5 ml/1 tsp vanilla essence (extract)
5 ml/1 tsp lemon juice

Place the apricots in a dish with 60 ml/4 tbsp of the water. Cover with clingfilm (plastic wrap) and slit it twice to allow steam to escape. Cook on Full for 8–9 minutes until the fruit is tender. Transfer to a food processor or blender and work to a purée with another 60 ml/4 tbsp of the water. Transfer to a 900 ml/1½ pt/3¾ cup bowl with the sugar. Mix the cornflour smoothly with the remaining water. Add to the purée in the bowl. Cook, uncovered, on Full for 2½–3½ minutes, whisking every 30 seconds, until the mixture has thickened and is clear and bubbling gently. Stir in the vanilla and lemon juice and use cold.

Home-made Caramel Sauce

Serves 4

50 g/2 oz/¼ cup dark soft brown sugar
30 ml/2 tbsp cold water
15 ml/1 tbsp boiling water

Put the sugar and cold water into a measuring jug or bowl. Cook, uncovered, on Full for 2 minutes until boiling, watching carefully in case it starts to burn. Remove from the microwave and stir in the boiling water. Use hot as an ice cream topping or for Crème Caramel.

Egg Custard Sauce

Serves 4–6

A golden, glowing sauce, bliss over sweets like Summer Fruit Mould, steamed puddings, stewed fruits, even trifle.

600 ml/1 pt/2½ cups full-cream milk or half milk and half single (light) cream
10 ml/2 tsp cornflour (cornstarch)
15 ml/1 tbsp cold water
4 large eggs
45 ml/3 tbsp caster (superfine) sugar
5 ml/1 tsp vanilla essence (extract)

Pour the milk into a 1.25 litre/2¼ pt/5½ cup measuring jug and heat, uncovered, on Full for 2 minutes. Place the flour in a 1.25 litre/2¼ pt/5½ cup bowl and mix smoothly with the water. Break in the eggs, then add the sugar. Whisk until smooth, then gradually blend in the hot milk. Cook, uncovered, on Full for 5–5½ minutes, whisking every minute, until the sauce clings to the spatula or wooden spoon used for whisking. Mix in the vanilla essence.

Flavoured Egg Custard Sauce

Serves 4–6

Prepare as for Egg Custard Sauce, but substitute rum, sherry, almond or rose essence (extract) for the vanilla essence.

Lemon or Orange Custard

Serves 4–6

Prepare as for Egg Custard Sauce, but substitute 10 ml/2 tsp finely grated orange or lemon peel for the vanilla essence.

Brandy Sauce

Serves 4

Traditionally served on Christmas Pudding, also for mince pies.

25 g/1 oz/2 tbsp butter or margarine
30 ml/2 tbsp plain (all-purpose) flour
300 ml/½ pt/1¼ cups warmed milk
25–30 ml/1½–2 tbsp caster (superfine) sugar
25–30 ml/1½–2 tbsp brandy

Put the butter or margarine in a 900 ml/1½ pt/3¾ cup bowl. Melt, uncovered, on Defrost for 30–45 seconds. Stir in the flour. Cook on Full for 30 seconds. Gradually blend in the milk. Cook, uncovered, on Full for 4–5 minutes, beating every minute, until thickened and smooth. Mix in the sugar and cook, uncovered, on Full for 30 seconds. Stir in the brandy and serve.

Rum Sauce

Serves 4

Prepare as for Brandy Sauce, but substitute rum for the brandy.

Orange Sauce

Serves 4

An elusively scented sauce for any kind of light steamed pudding.

Prepare as for Brandy Sauce, but add 5 ml/1 tsp finely grated orange rind with the flour and substitute 15 ml/1 tbsp orange flower water for the brandy.

Sticky Toffee Sauce

Serves 4

Setting chewily on impact with ice cream, this is a heavenly sauce for any kind of sundae.

50 g/2 oz/¼ cup butter
40 g/1½ oz light soft brown sugar
50 g/2 oz marshmallows
15 ml/1 tbsp milk

Put all the ingredients in a 1.75 litre/3 pt/7½ cup bowl (the large size is necessary because the mixture rises as it cooks). Melt, uncovered, on Defrost for 2 minutes. Stir thoroughly. Heat on Full for a further 2½ minutes, stirring carefully three times. Use straight away as this sauce sets quickly.

Fresh Raspberry Sauce

Serves 4

Fresh and fragrant, a superior summer sauce for sundaes based on nectarines or peaches and vanilla ice cream.

10 ml/2 tsp cornflour (cornstarch)
150 ml/¼ pt/2/3 cup single (light) cream
30 ml/2 tbsp caster (superfine) sugar
225 g/8 oz/2 cups fresh raspberries, carefully rinsed
15 ml/1 tbsp cherry brandy

Put the cornflour in a 1.5 litre/2½ pt/6 cup bowl and mix smoothly with some of the cream. Stir in the remaining cream with the sugar and half the raspberries. Cook, uncovered, on Full for 4 minutes, stirring every minute. Fold in the remaining raspberries with the cherry brandy. Serve warm.

Chocolate Honey Raisin Sauce

Serves 6–8

Wonderful over coffee ice cream or orange sorbet.

50 g/2 oz/1/3 cup raisins
15 ml/1 tbsp boiling water
100 g/3½ oz plain (semi-sweet) chocolate
25 g/1 oz/2 tbsp butter
30 ml/2 tbsp single (light) cream
30 ml/2 tbsp thick honey
5 ml/1 tsp vanilla essence (extract)

Soak the raisins in the boiling water. Break up the chocolate and place in a small bowl with the butter. Melt, uncovered, on Defrost for about 3½ minutes. Stir in the cream, honey and vanilla. Heat, uncovered, on Full for 30–40 seconds. Drain the raisins and stir in.

www.ingramcontent.com/pod-product-compliance
Lightning Source LLC
Chambersburg PA
CBHW071821080526
44589CB00012B/871